BEATING DIABETES

THE LOW-CARB WAY

Dr Chris Barclay

STA BOOKS

ISBN: 978-0-9933957-6-5

PUBLISHED BY STA BOOKS
www.spencerthomasassociates.com

Cover Image © Shelley Nott

About the book

Welcome to Planet Diabetes

Type-2 Diabetes and overweight/obesity are now the most common long-term medical conditions in the western world. Yet two generations ago, they hardly existed. What has changed? The simple answer is that it's our diets. When the low-fat era began in the 1980s, we needed something to fill our plates and those somethings were sugary and starchy foods; carbohydrates, in other words. The dramatic and unprecedented rise of dietary carbs neatly coincided with the very moment obesity and diabetes began to explode in our societies, perhaps one of the greatest unintended consequences in modern history. Can anything be done? Yes! Should we just leave it to our doctors and dieticians to manage our inevitable decline? No! This happened on their watch. Instead, why not cut the carbs and try to reverse diabesity? *Beating Diabetes* explains how and why this happened and, vitally and precisely, what to do about it.

About the author

Dr Chris Barclay is a GP and medical writer. His special interest in diet and health began with a chance encounter; a patient told him how he had lost weight by cutting out carbohydrate foods. Dr Barclay has researched the subject ever since. He was principal investigator for the ISAIAH Project, a diet trial in pre-diabetic patients. His conclusion – processed carbs, starchy foods and sugar are the problem; they are driving our diabesity epidemic. In *Beating Diabetes,* Dr Barclay presents compelling and persuasive evidence translated into a practical and effective plan. Dr Barclay has written extensively for several medical magazines. He is the principal writer for MaPPs, a medicines information website. He worked for many years as a GP in Sheffield and more recently in Aldeburgh, Suffolk, UK. Dr Barclay is an Ambassador for the Public Health Collaboration, a UK charity that promotes health through real-food and low-carb dining.

Disclaimer

The opinions expressed in this book Dr Barclay's personal views. They are the beliefs that now guide his own day-to-day eating and dining habits. He shares these opinions and beliefs for general information purposes only. They are not intended to be and should not be, relied upon as medical advice. No doctor/patient relationship exists. The publisher and author are not responsible for any health need that may require medical advice or supervision. The use of any information and opinions expressed in this book is done so at the reader's own risk. They are not intended to be a substitute for professional medical attention, advice, diagnosis, or treatment. This is especially so for anyone on any prescribed medication and, in particular, medications used in the treatment of diabetes. Users should not ignore or delay obtaining medical advice for any medical condition they may have. If you have any medical or health conditions or problems, or if you require advice, you should contact a qualified medical, dietary or other appropriate professional.

Bottom line: Speak to your doctor before changing your diet and, if you are on any medication, do not change anything before consultation with your doctor.

Acknowledgements

Perhaps the person I have most reason to thank is 'that patient' (he knows who he is) who told me how he had lost weight after reading a book called *Dine Out and Lose Weight*[1]. He just did what it said. That encounter nudged me into a journey of discovery and into the realms of nutritional heresy. Nigel Mathers, then Professor of General Practice and Primary Care at Sheffield's School of Medicine, continued the process. He became my intellectual midwife, birthing me into the outer fringes of academia; a strange land I inhabited but briefly. While I was under his wing, we devised a scientific study to test out what I had already come to name the ISAIAH Project[2].

Our collaboration was profitable and Nigel takes much credit for fanning my flames of curiosity. Nigel also helped recruit a team to investigate the ISAIAH approach. Each member deserves thanks for their suggestions, support and contributions to the pilot study testing out a programme in General Practice. So, thank you to Sharon Hart, Maria Platts, Dr Robert Glendenning, Professor Peter Marsh, Dr Jenny Freeman, Alex Bonnett, Nettie Goldsworthy, Ann Wright and most especially Dr Kim Edwards (previously Proctor). I must also give especial thanks to the longsuffering doctors and staff, friends and former colleagues, at the Nethergreen Surgery, Sheffield, for putting up with the intrusion of ISAIAH into their already busy lives. Nigel deserves extra thanks for inviting me back to lecture on the Obituary of a Randomised Controlled Trial to visiting post-graduate students. Actually, the obituary was premature. ISAIAH still lives and breathes and has become *Beating Diabetes*.

The years after publication of the pilot trial were filled with the excitement of discovering that I was not the only heretic out there. As a matter of fact, the principles of *Beating Diabetes* have been around for nearly two centuries in various guises and under different names. It turns out that a lot of people have been shouting 'The emperor has no clothes' at official diets around the world for a very long time. The writers who (totally unbeknown to them) particularly guided my thinking and whose scholarship I gratefully acknowledge include, in no particular order: Gary Taubes, Charles Clark, Michael Pollan, Denise Minger, Nina Teicholz, Robert Lustig, Zoë Harcombe, Sarah Hallberg, Malcolm Kendrick, David Ludwig, Jason Fung. There are many others. Professor Aseem Malhotra deserves particular thanks, not just for his groundbreaking myth-busting work on what actually causes heart disease, what constitutes a truly healthy diet and the role of physical activity in health, but for generously writing the foreword to *Beating Diabetes*. I feel so privileged that he agreed to helpand astounded at how quickly he responded.

Particular respect is due to a handful of British dietary giants from the mid-nineteenth to the twentieth centuries: William Banting, Thomas 'Peter' Cleeve, John Yudkin and Richard Mackarness. Their influence was never as great as they deserved. The steamroller that is the 'Official Diet' rolled over and squashed them. Today their names will be known to but a few. They were, each in their various ways, heroes, in my view. Only latterly have I added Dr Wolfgang Lutz to my person dietary pantheon.

This book started out as an enjoyable escape and a way of organising my thoughts by committing them to paper; a sort of personal cognitive therapy. Exploring insights that contradict the current nutritional paradigm has been rather time-consuming. So, both thanks and apologies to my wonderful wife, Bev, for permitting me to spend hours and hours reading, thinking, writing and then boring her with the fruits of the process. Thanks to Rebecca Baker for so expertly (and gently) editing the manuscript. Thanks to Sue Nicholson, who didn't look bored when I explained what I was doing and went on to do a bit of literary matchmaking. We do say that whatever the question might be, someone in our village will either know the answer or have a connection. This time it was Sue and her friend Fiona. So, thanks to my agent and publisher, Fiona Spencer Thomas, for that lovely lunch in Pimlico and bravely taking me on and being another midwife on the journey

Notes:

1. Dine out and lose weight. Michel Montignac. Montignac Publishing (UK); 2nd Revised edition (1 Jan. 1996).
2. **ISAIAH.** An acronym that stands for Insulin Sensitivity And Its Applications to Health.

Contents

Foreword by Dr Aseem Malhotra

In the 1950s a man from Minnesota in the United States had a big idea, an idea he called The Diet-Heart Hypothesis. In a moment of misguided inspiration, he decided that heart attacks just had to be the result of consuming too much fat. No sooner had he had his big idea than he began to search diligently for evidence to support it; and of course, he found it. However, by looking only for favourable facts, he committed one of the Cardinal Sins of medical research. The well-established and indeed only safe way to determine the truth would have been to have tried to *disprove* his hypothesis; if it cannot be disproved then perhaps it might be right.

This one man was blessed with a phenomenal capacity for hard work, but sadly he was also cursed with an intolerant and bullying personality. To cut a very long story short, by the mid 1980s and in the face of firm evidence to the contrary, low-fat diets became the new-normal for official advice on both sides of the Atlantic. The Diet-Heart Hypothesis became dietary gospel.

The problems with this new low-fat approach were twofold. Firstly, fat (even saturated fat) never did and still does not cause heart disease, quite the contrary in fact. Secondly, when all that fat got scraped off our plates we had to replace it with something. Those somethings were processed sugary and starchy foods, the sort of foods that have now become 'normal' staple fodder for much of the population. They said low-fat; we got high-carb. That, in a nutshell, is how we have come to base most of every meal we now eat on refined processed carbohydrate foods 'low-fat' foods. The unintended consequence of this low-fat/high-carb approach has been the epidemics of diabetes and obesity.

This new high-carb regime was a gift to Big-Food businesses. With their generous subsidies and economies of scale our tables began to heave with mounds of potato wedges, pizzas, pasta salads, rice dishes, couscous, cakes, bagels, confectionery, croissants and sugary sodas.

We now get all-day sugar and all-day grazing. Tsunamis of sugar wash into us from that first fruit juice of the day till the final fridge-raid before bed; and it is killing us.

These new high-carb diet guidelines were also a gift for the Big Pharmaceutical businesses. The more ill and fat we got, the more the money poured in. The treatment guidelines they endorsed were great for an army of healthcare experts and medical academics whose tsunami-surfing careers have flourished. Welcome to *Planet Diabetes*; we are in hell of a mess.

With this in mind I found Dr Chris Barclay's important new book *Beating Diabetes the low-carb way* a breath of fresh air. His book is a well-organised compendium of the practical life-changing advice he has been giving his own patients for the last twenty years; advice based on what he calls *clinical wisdom*. In it he has weighed and sifted the sciences of nutrition and diabetes (and its unfortunate sibling, obesity) and presented his findings in the form of down to earth, real-life, real-food advice. In academic terms *Beating Diabetes* is a work of translation in that it has gathered evidence from a wide range of sources and nicely re-packaged it all in a readable and clearly understandable way. It's a toolkit for mending bodies afflicted with diabetes.

If my own book *The Pioppi Diet: A 21-day Lifestyle Plan*, written with Donal O'Neill, addresses the questions - what to do about and how to avoid, coronary heart disease, Chris's is a what to do about and how to avoid, Type-2 diabetes. Our books are in fact two sides of the very same coin. We both sing (loudly) from the same hymn sheet. We are both deeply concerned that the well of published studies from which we draw our 'evidence' has been poisoned by vested interest, overblown claims and, all too often, disseminated without question by a naïve press. We are both considered by the establishment to be medical heretics because we both keep shouting 'the emperor wears no clothes'. In the face of so much avoidable suffering and unnecessary medication, we can do nothing else.

As Chris says "all diets work for someone; no diet works for everyone" but if you are overweight or have Type-2 diabetes, particularly if your diabetes is in its early stages, *Beating Diabetes* could be very good news for you by offering a leg up out of the low-fat/low-cal rut of failure.

Sadly, the irresistible tide of evidence and the numerous success stories that are out there in plain sight, are yet to have any significant impact on our conflicted Official Diet experts. Nor have these changed the default and usually unconsidered mindset of most medical doctors and their fellow healthcare colleagues; at least, not yet. So, why not give a copy to your doctor or specialist diabetes nurse. The tide is turning. Let's pray that it is soon.

Dr Aseem Malhotra - Consultant Cardiologist

Conventions used in this book

1. **Diabetes/Diabesity**. This is a book about diabesity; the twins that are Type-2 Diabetes and Obesity. They are just two sides of a single coin, linked to a single common cause. So, when you see the word diabetes used in this book, you should take it to mean Type-2 Diabetes unless it is explicitly stated otherwise. You should also understand the word diabetes to be something that is often almost identical to and co-terminus with overweight and obesity. The remedy for both diabetes and overweight/obesity presented here is one and the same because, for most people, they have one and the same basic dietary cause. So, if your particular interest is more about overweight/obesity, you can assume that in this book diabetes means much the same thing.

2. **Sugar.** The word sugar has many meanings. It can mean glucose (the sugar found in the bloodstream) or sucrose (the stuff we stir into our tea and sprinkle on strawberries). It has other meanings too but, like Humpty Dumpty, I have used the term sugar to mean precisely what I want it to mean[1]. At times it will signify sucrose/table sugar and at others, glucose/blood sugar. It should be pretty obvious as you read which is which. Where I have been technically imprecise, it has simply been to help with readability and to keep jargon to the bare minimum.

3. **Cure/Remission.** The word *cure* is an odd one. The dictionary would suggest a remedy or intervention that restores health. In real medical practice, things are never quite so black and white; we medics live forever in a world of shades of grey. We talk of cure rates and relative estimates of your chance of benefiting and almost never in terms of an absolute guarantee. So, what does a cure mean in this book? Well, it means a way to try and reverse a problem. For some people that may mean a complete cure. Others may see a degree of remission, an improvement in weight or sugar control, or perhaps a reduction in medication

requirement. Of course, if you are the sort of person who got diabetes in the first place, then it stands to reason that it could all come back again if a successful dietary change is just temporary. If you go back to high-carb processed fodder, you're likely to have to go back to your doctor too, sooner rather than later. Having said that, biology is inherently variable and how we respond and react to change can never be predicted with certainty but hey, what's the alternative?

Notes:

1. It was Humpty Dumpty who said 'When I use a word it means just what I choose it to mean.' From *Through the Looking Glass* by Lewis Carroll.

Part 1

Introduction

Chapter 1 – Welcome to planet diabetes

Status quo, you know, is Latin for

'the mess we're in'

Ronald Regan[1]

'If you have Type-2 Diabetes, tough. You are stuck with it. If you are lucky, we may slow it down for you but it never goes away' or so conventional medical wisdom would have us believe. It is wrong. This is not wisdom. This is folly.

Type-2 Diabetes, especially in its early stages, can be reversed. For many, reversing diabetes is devastatingly simple. Diabetes, you see, happens when the body has lost its ability to handle sugary and starchy foods efficiently; basically carbohydrates. Someone with diabetes who continues to eat these types of foods will usually find that their condition gets worse. It is not called 'sugar-diabetes' for nothing. If that person chooses to cut out those foods, or at least cut down on them significantly, they will almost always find their diabetes problem improves. Some may even enter a total remission and, if they stick with the lifestyle change, they could achieve a permanent remission; a cure. It is unlikely your doctor or nurse will tell you this and the nation's Official experts won't tell you this either. This is the mess we're in.

High blood sugar levels, you see, are not the *cause* of diabetes, high blood sugars are the *result* of diabetes. Diabetes causes blood sugar levels to run high, not the other way around. In the early stages of Type-2 Diabetes, the body has far too much insulin going around. This is the opposite of what we see in Type-1 (the one that often starts in childhood), where there is a complete absence of insulin. Type-2 Diabetes is, at least initially, a condition with a gross insulin excess; too much insulin, produced in response to a high-carb diet. Dig just a little deeper and you will discover that, behind the sugar problems of diabetes, something else is going on; something called insulin resistance.

Insulin excess and insulin resistance are main causes of diabetes, indeed you could say that they *are* diabetes; the raised blood sugar level is merely an effect. So, right from the outset, please bear in mind that if someone wants to reverse their diabetes, they need to focus on insulin levels and insulin resistance rather than what their blood sugar, or even that longer term measure of blood glucose, your HbA1c levels, happens to be[2]. They are important but only as a part of the whole story. Straighten out the insulin problem and they generally straighten out their blood sugar problem too. Medical management, however, usually focuses just on getting blood sugar levels down, totally ignoring the underlying the insulin resistance problem. It's looking down the wrong end of the telescope. It is obsessed with the effects of diabetes and ignores its driving cause. As Ronald Regan might have said, 'This is the mess we're in.'

Worse still, today our normal everyday medical approach to diabetes has become part of the unfolding disaster, precisely because it focuses on blood sugar levels to the exclusion of everything else. The aim of orthodox medical treatment of diabetes is to achieve *euglycaemia* (Latin for a normal glucose level in the blood). Correcting the underlying insulin problem is not the point; it is not even on the agenda and never has been. The usual medical approach only sees the consequences of diabetes and ignores its cause (Figure 1.1) and, as a result, all its efforts (drugs, basically) zoom in on your blood glucose and HbA1 levels to the exclusion of almost everything else (Figure 1.2). This is, in my view, folly. Imagine going to your dentist with a tooth abscess only to be given a painkiller. No doubt it would help with the pain but it would do nothing for the underlying problem or the abscess. Now imagine going back because your pain has got worse and you have started with a fever, only to be given a stronger painkiller. Imagine if antibiotics or a dental extraction to cure the infection were never on offer. You just got your symptoms treated while the fire in your tooth raged on.

Figure 1.1 The journey into Type-2 Diabetes and its consequences

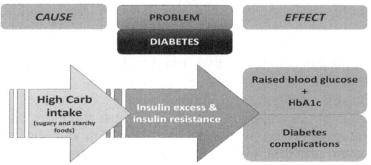

Figure 1.1 Type-2 Diabetes is a dietary disorder, mainly caused by sugary and starchy carb foods. It is, at least in its early stages, the combination of insulin excess secretion and insulin resistance. Knowing this allows you to see that, what most people consider diabetes to be is, i.e. raised blood glucose levels as well as the many complications of diabetes, are in facts effects and not causes. Most treatments target these effects rather than the true underlying problem, let alone its cause. In long-standing diabetes, the pancreas fails and the insulin levels drop.

Well, sadly, that is how modern medicine generally treats diabetes. Reversing insulin excess and insulin resistance, the twin drivers of diabetes, are not its goals. Most doctors and specialist nurses view diabetes as a chronic (long-term) inevitably progressive (gets worse and worse) condition caused by high blood sugar levels. Reversing diabetes, in their view, is a joke and a sick one at that. In all likelihood, you will rarely hear the words 'excess insulin' and 'insulin resistance' from your doctors and nurses. Just to make things worse, our modern drugs are not designed to reverse your diabetes either. Their job, like those painkillers for a dental abscess, is just to ease things awhile. This is the mess we're in.

Now, you may know that one of insulin's main jobs is to

deal with blood sugar, or glucose, to be precise; insulin brings blood glucose levels down after meals. If someone eats foods that do not drive up glucose levels, or if they go a step further and have short periods of fasting too, their insulin levels will drop. In fact, they will drop rapidly, on Day-1. If they do these things regularly, their insulin resistance will respond as well. The end result? They will have started their *Beating Diabetes* journey. You see diabetes is a condition caused by diet and the only true remedy is a dietary one. If their diabetes-causing diet does not change their diabetes will almost always progress, although the drugs may slow that progress down a bit.

Unfortunately, those with diabetes will probably not have been told this. They will probably not have been told that they have a carbohydrate-caused and a carbohydrate-driven condition. They probably won't have been told that all that insulin is their body desperately trying to protect itself from their dietary choices. Worse, they will almost certainly actively be encouraged to continue eating the very foods that caused their diabetes in the first place: sugary and starchy foods. The Official guidance on managing diabetes is to base every meal on diabetes-causing foods – food like bread, potato, rice, pasta and fruit. Then, when that dietary advice fails, as it almost always does, the only remaining tool Dr Diabetes has in his box is medication. Yes, they will be given drugs to cope with their diet. Reversing the condition is never on the agenda. Instead they will be medically managed. They are diabetic so, obviously, you need anti-diabetic drugs. They will become a citizen of Planet Diabetes. This is the mess we're in.

So, what is this book all about? Well, it is mostly about three things.

Firstly, it looks very critically at our Official dietary guidance and reveals how it actually causes people to develop diabetes. When the fog of misinformation clears, you will be able to see for yourself the whole diet-diabetes thing quite clearly. The solution will then be obvious.

Secondly, it reveals how Official dietary guidance is not

only a major contributory cause of diabetes but it actually makes diabetes worse. Shovelling more and more carbs into a body wracked by the carb-intolerance disorder that is diabetes just makes no sense at all.

Third and most importantly, because Official dietary guidance is a major contributor to the diabetes problem (and because the food industry cannot be relied upon to provide healthy nourishment either) I explore precisely how diabetes can be reversed and how, for some, a complete reversal may even be possible.

I am sorry to say that for most of us the only person who can be relied upon to turn things around is the patient. This book is their toolkit. It tells them things they will almost certainly not hear from most health professionals. Instead, it enables them to understand and then implement their own personal *Beating Diabetes* plan. As someone once said, 'Reversing' diabetes starts with ignoring the guidelines'[3]. This really is the mess we're in.

It does have to be said that a low-carb approach will not work for everyone. As a matter of fact, nothing ever does work for everyone but these diet changes do work for a lot of people and maybe for most with diabetes. They also work for most people heading rapidly in the direction of diabetes, particularly those with pre-diabetes or who are overweight. The good news is that it is possible to re-route oneself away from that whole *diabesity* thing and turn back on to the highway to health[2].

Figure 1.2 Where low-carb diet change and medicines are targetted

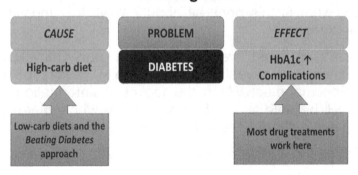

Figure 1.2 Almost all medicines used to treat diabetes target the effects of the condition. Metformin is an exception in that it reduces insulin resistance (part of the problem). If carbs are not reduced then in effect Metformin and all those other medicines are working to reduce the adverse effect of a high-carb diet; using drugs to treat your food in other words.

My mission here is to tell you the hows and whys and whats to do. Actually, nothing in this book is new. All I have done is to collect as many useful strands of information from as far and wide as I could, then knitted them all together. Nor is the low-carb approach unique; many people today are busy reinventing the wheel for themselves. In fact, wheel-reinventing about diabetes and obesity has been going on for well over half a century but the wheel-smashers have been just as busy. There are now extensive low-carb/healthy-fat and fasting communities out there and beating diabetes is one of the many things they do. So, this is a work of translation; translating the established science already out there in plain view, into a plan that works for Type-2 Diabetes and pre-diabetes. Much of it will be news to you. Indeed, much of it might well be news to my health professional brothers and sisters too. If you are eager to know (right now) what your problem is and what are its solutions, well, in a nutshell – here goes…

Our Official dietary guidance, the guidance that has now become pretty well universal across Europe, North America and Australasia for two generations says:

'Cut fat, cut saturated-fat, cut calories. Fill up on starchy foods like bread, pasta and potato at every meal. Oh and, by the way, eat plenty of fruit and veg'. What those of us in the low-carb community say is:

'Cut those carbs, celebrate and enjoy the fat in your diet and perhaps consider being creative about regular short fasts. Oh and, by the way, go easy on the fruit as it is in fact high-fructose tree-candy.'

So, if you want to clue up on carbs, read on. If you think fat is your foe, read on. You are wrong, it isn't. Fat is your friend. If you think fasting is foolish and grazing is great, you really need to read on. If you think five, eight or even ten-a-day is the key to healthful bliss, read on. If you believe carbs are essential, read on. They are not. Most carbs equal insulin and, for many of us, our all-day-insulin habit (the new normal) is _the_ cause of diabetes and much else besides. So, just read on.

The long march to Diabesity

Humans have walked this planet for almost 250,000 years and for almost all that time, we were hunter-gatherers. The range of foods we subsisted on during those many years was wide and diverse, dependent on habitat and climate. Our ancestors hunted for meat, poultry and fish and they gathered leaves, nuts, roots, berries and fruit. Many followed their food supplies nomadically.

But around 10,000 years ago, something new happened, a revolutionary dietary change swept across the globe. Somewhere, probably in the present-day Levant, we began to farm. Actually, farming started independently very soon afterwards around the world. We cleared the ground, made fields, tilled soil, planted seeds and grew crops; mainly coarse grains at first. It was not a coincidence that around that same time the first organised settlements were established. We built towns and the farms around them fed us and it was these farms that first introduced significant quantities of starchy grains and rough flour into humanity's diet. They gave us something we had never seen before, something we have been in love with ever since: bread. The introduction of starchy flour was an agricultural revolution and perhaps, after the discovery that fire could be used to improve food, the first of humankind's many diet transformations.

A pastoral revolution happened a millennium or more later. The first cattle, sheep and goats were herded together and domestication was bred into them. This gave us easy access to meat and dairy foods. Before this, the only milk a human ever tasted was from its mother's breast. We soon learned to make cheese and butter and, with plant husbandry and improvement, we developed a gastronomy. However, it took until the eighteenth and nineteenth centuries and the industrial revolution, for another of our great dietary transformations. The wind and water milling of corn and wheat into wholegrain flours was replaced with engine-powered devices, ones that could efficiently separate the starchy flour from the fibrous husk and the germ; we got white flour and we got it in industrial quantities. Machines were also built to purify cane sugar and Africa was shamefully plundered for souls to work the plantations. Later the invention of industrial sugar-beet processing allowed the damp and muddy fields of northern Europe to make sugar too. Refined flour and refined sugar burst into out kitchens and suddenly became essential staples in our daily diet.

In more recent times, we have witnessed another agricultural revolution, the emergence of a vast global system that moves raw ingredients around in unimaginably huge quantities. Farmers may have given us agriculture, but economists, speculators and multinational food producers have long since taken over. Global agribusiness now feeds the world.

Sugar and spice and all things nice?

Food scientists tell us that there are just three major and three minor food types. Fats, proteins and carbohydrates are the majors; vitamins, minerals and fibre the minors. Actually, some would argue that alcohol should now be considered a major food type too (see Appendix 5 for details of why this might be the case and why it is particularly important to those with diabetes or weight problems). These days you might also tack on all those non-nutrient additives, preservatives and mouthfeel enhancers, etcetera, that our food manufacturers sneak into their products. Anyway, of the three major food types, our hunter-gatherer ancestors relied almost exclusively on just two; fats and proteins. They did consume carbs, but in smaller amounts than we do today and their carbs were the stringy unimproved types with little starch or sugar in them. Blood sugar surges after eating were both modest and infrequent back then.

Carbs come in three forms; sugars, starches and fibre. The only sugars our ancestors ever had access to were fruits and berries in season, honey if and when they could get it, maple syrup perhaps if they lived in North America and, of course, the special sugars present in breast milk. Starches featured even less frequently on their menus, perhaps from the occasional chewed root, seed or grain, or from the special form of starch found in liver meat: glycogen.

Before farming took off, sugary and starchy foods were only consumed occasionally and guess what? The need for hunter-gatherers to secrete matching surges of insulin, (our sugar-control hormone) were both modest and occasional too. For them the sugar-hit happened just a few times a year. For us modern humans, blood sugar surges typically happen many times every single day. If hunter-gatherers had a problem it was how to keep their blood sugar levels up. Today it is different; our problem is how to keep sugar levels down. Hunter-gatherers motored along quite nicely on sugar from food and sugar made from the glycogen stores within the body. They relied far more, almost exclusively so, on that other major fuel our bodies run very nicely on – fat. Our hunter-gatherer ancestors were smart multi-fuel machines. Today we rely almost exclusively on just one single power source, glucose-sugar from the food we eat. Unlike glycogen-sugar and fat, all the food-derived sugars and starches oblige us to secrete insulin. As a matter of fact, insulin is also secreted in response to protein foods like meat, eggs and fish but at a very much lower level than those seen when eating modern processed carbohydrate foods. Fatty foods do not cause any insulin release at all.

It's the insulin, stupid! - *Robert Lustig*[4]

Why, you may be wondering, are the first pages of a

dietary advice book for people with Type-2 Diabetes majoring on chemistry and ancient history and not recipes? The answer is simple. Getting some understanding of how our biology works with various food types is a golden key and that key can open a door to understanding diabetes. Unlike our hunter-gatherer forebears, typical modern eating habits, the ones promoted these days in all the Official dietary guidance, cause tsunamis of sugar to surge into our bodies. In human history terms, this is new. The inevitable consequence is that we are obliged to match those sugar surges with tsunamis of insulin. This too is new in human biology. Of course, insulin's major job is to bring sugar levels down but insulin is also the body's hormone of storage. It lowers blood sugar levels by transforming sugar into fat and storing it. Insulin came in very handy for those hunter-gatherers when they came across a rare sugary feast, like honey or fruit. It allowed them to convert the sugars into fat. Insulin is very good at doing this, as that is what it is for. Insulin allowed them to store up that energy in anticipation of future lean times, like winter. For them, collecting honey was a dangerous business and fruit was never in season for long. When the fruit and honey were consumed, our ancestors may have weighed a pound or two more but, unlike today, they may well have had to endure times of hunger. That stock of stored energy might then have made the difference between life and death. Insulin made them a little fatter during those rare but welcome sugar surges. It converted it to fat and pumped it into fat cells and while insulin was around, it blocked the fat cells from releasing it. It's the insulin-carb combo that makes you fat but it is insulin that keeps you fat too. That's what we evolved to do and way back then it made perfect sense.

Today it is different. We get sugar/glucose surges all the time. We get it from our fruit juice and cereal at breakfast, that mid-morning pastry with coffee, our sandwich or wrap for lunch, those biscuits with tea, that pasta, pizza, potato or rice meal for dinner, those naughty-but-nice crisps or crackers for supper, to that last lingering after-supper morsel of toast before bed. While we are awake, we are rarely far from eating starchy foods that wash sugar into our bodies, even if we have not consumed a single grain of the sweet white stuff. The result? Our body chemistry is dominated by insulin in a way never before seen in human history or, for that matter in primate history either. Insulin is now present directing our body chemistry the wrong way from dawn to well beyond dusk.

That, in a nutshell, is why many of us get so fat. That is why so many of us stay fat and that is why fat and calorie restriction diets so often fail. Overweight/obesity is mostly a hormone-driven problem. It never was a simple calorie-excess problem. Sadly, that hormonal imbalance is why so many of us get diabetes and its devastating complications too. That's why so many people with diabetes are told to keep taking medications (to treat the effects of their food). Insulin excess is the body's natural response to our modern unnatural diets and that obligatory insulin excess is driving our diabetes and obesity epidemics.

So why are we constantly being told to eat the very sugary and starchy carbs that fatten us and make so many of us ill? Why are the overweight advised to base one third of their diet on the very carbs that are guaranteed, through the insulin surges they evoke, to prevent weight loss? Why are diabetics being advised to eat even more of the very stuff that made them diabetic in the first place and then given drugs to control the effects of their Official carb-heavy diet advice? Why are we now expecting people with diabetes to take medication to offset the effects of their food? The answer, I suspect, is a combination of three things: something called the diet-heart hypothesis, understandable human inertia and vested interest. Group-think is a difficult thing to overcome.

Until the late 1970s, it was well understood that sweet (sugars) and farinaceous foods (starchy things like potato, rice and flour-based products) were particularly fattening. Dr Spock, the twentieth century guru of child health and development, cautioned against them because, as it was well known, they made children obese[5]. In the second half of the twentieth century, things changed abruptly in the United States. Something called 'the diet-heart hypothesis' was born and, like a cuckoo, it threw every other dietary approach out of the nest. Although it was only a theory, an unproven idea in other words, it was vigorously promoted as if it were absolute truth. It swept away everything else before it.

In the 1950s and 60s, there was panic in the US about the number of affluent middle-aged men dropping dead from heart attacks. The diet-heart hypothesis insisted that heart attacks were being caused by too much fat in the diet. The arguments made at the time seemed compelling to those in authority but it turned out they were wrong. Natural fat in the diet did not cause heart disease then and it does not do so now. There is no good evidence that it does and plenty that it does not. Politics and vested interests kicked in and prevailed and America embarked on an uncharted voyage across an ocean of low-fat everything. Opposing views and opinions, no matter how scientifically valid, were squashed mercilessly. It functioned like a sort of dietary McCarthyism.

A few years later in the early 1980s, the UK's Official dietary advisors, like sheep (or perhaps lemmings), obediently fell in line and they too launched their nations on the low-fat regime. It was from these very years that obesity and diabetes rates took a sudden and unexpected lurch upwards and they have been climbing ever since. You see, when fat was stripped out, sugars and starches got added in. We had to eat something after all and, after removing fat, adding extra sugars and starches and often more salt too, was the only way to make things taste good.

Why, you may ask, are your doctor, nurse, dietician, Government Minister for Health, the relevant national campaigning charities, Uncle Tom Cobley and all, not telling you this? You may well ask. Partly it may be because two generations of health professionals have been brought up on the low-fat/lo-cal regime and the diet-heart hypothesis.

That is all they have been fed for forty years and their brains and palates know nothing different. To them it is unthinkable that the dietary-fat heart theory could be wrong. After all it makes perfect sense to them. It is a simple solution to a complex problem that ticks all the boxes. It never occurs to them that the low-fat/low-cal approach could be in error. To them, obesity is simply an imbalance in calorie accountancy and fat being calorie-dense is the obvious culprit. Compounding their error, they also adhere to the belief that fat in the diet causes heart attacks. It doesn't.

A small phrase to look out for, like a nasty little bindweed that should be pulled up on sight, is 'a balanced diet'. Regard anyone you hear uttering this piece of Orwellian *newspeak* with the greatest suspicion[6]. It tends to mean whatever the speaker wants it to mean and it comes with a subtext of 'I know best'. In general, it appears to mean a 5-a-day diet that is low-fat, low-cal and includes the food items that grace the Eatwell Guide pictures devised by Public Health England (PHE) or The US Dietary Guidelines for Americans. By the standards of PHE and the Eatwell Guide, some of the healthiest populations the world has ever seen appear to have seriously unbalanced diets.

Take for example those remaining Inuit peoples of the high Arctic who maintain a traditional eating habit. They get by on a diet of seal, fish, whale skin and walrus very nicely. Some also enjoy a delicacy known as stink-fish; raw fish that has been allowed to rot for a while. It is, I am informed, an acquired taste. These people rarely see a plant, let alone eat one and they do not have any dairy foods. Theirs was and, in a few places, still is a very high-fat, very low-carb diet; a diet almost devoid of sugars and almost without starchy carbs either; no wholegrains and no fruit, not even a satsuma for Christmas, although they may gather berries in season. Nevertheless, it was a diet upon which they thrived. Obesity, diabetes, dementia, cancer and heart disease were almost unheard of. In recent years, the eating habits of most of the Canadian Inuit peoples have been 'civilised' and they have become more North American, more westernised, in other words more 'balanced'. As a result their health has suffered hugely. Diabetes and obesity are rampant. According to PHE, these people now have a balanced diet and yet they have never been so sick. Many on the other hand would contend that previously, when they lived on their so-called unbalanced high-fat diet, they had an amazingly balanced metabolism and great health. Now here's the rub. Things were in balance, not because of what they ate, rather it was because of what they did *not* eat. They did not eat sugary and starchy carbs or processed foods. Give me a truly balanced metabolism over an Officially balanced diet any day. Therein lies the simple road to healthy eating.

In the same way, overweight and obesity are mostly the signs (not the causes) of a disordered body chemistry. They are about glands and hormones, as my overweight patients often complained and now I believe many of them were right. The gland is the pancreas and the hormone is insulin. Over half a century ago, one enlightened physician said that [it is difficult to] store fat in the absence of insulin and you cannot release fat in its presence[7]. The weird thing is that you can explain this to health professionals. They can understand it and even believe it to be true but, almost every time, they remain unable to detach themselves from the 'dietary fat and gluttony is what makes you fat' paradigm. They are unable to see obesity for what it is; a hormonally driven metabolic disorder or, to put it more simply, a condition caused, dominated and driven by too much insulin. A neat psychological term for this inability to resolve the conflict between facts and beliefs is cognitive dissonance. This is an uncomfortable place to be. Most find it easier to just blame their patients. Let's face it, it is so much easier than confronting some very inconvenient truths. The irresistible forces of reality have not yet shifted the immovable object of orthodox belief.

Okay, let us revisit the opening questions. What is this book all about and who it for? Let me answer the second question first. This book is for me. It is my own personal healthy eating belief. I do not want to get Type-2 Diabetes, nor any of the other conditions driven by our modern carbo-centric food beliefs. I say this because I have been overweight and fear I could easily drift into diabetes myself. It is also for my own diabetic and pre-diabetic patients who wish to avoid getting ill and want to do something radical about it. I regularly discuss diet and lifestyle questions during consultations and this book is a collection of the evidence and wisdom I draw on during these clinical encounters. Thirdly, *Beating Diabetes* may also be a book for you to consider.

This book is about the dangers of sugar, starch and too much insulin and describes in a practical way what can be done about it. It is about how folk with diabetes or pre-diabetes can eat more healthily, more in tune with their body's chemistry and thereby reduce the risk of getting the so-called disease of Western civilisation. We live in confusing times. The range of views on what constitutes healthy eating is vast, contradictory sometimes, vitriolic at times, confusing certainly and, particularly on the internet, covertly tainted by vested interests. It is a mess and a dangerous one at that. My belief, for what it's worth, is that healthy eating should chime with the biology we have all inherited from our stone-age ancestors. So, like them, I enjoy a range and diversity of foods and I mimic their diets by keeping sugary and starchy foods to a minimum. They didn't have this choice but, sadly, we do. So, this is a book about low-carb dining. Oh, did you notice the 'D' word there; dine? It is not just what we eat that matters. *How* we eat is also important.

This book has four sections:

The first Introductory section is about the basics of 'How did I get diabetes', '…and what can I do about it?' Here you will find much about how we came to be a Diabetic Nation and, in a very practical sense, what can be done about it. I use the word cure occasionally and very advisedly. This is not the same thing as managing the problem. This section contains background essays for those of you who want to know more about *diabesity* (basically the diabetes and obesity epidemics)[8].

The second section is about how to actually beat diabetes. In Shop, Cook, Dine, Fast and Exercise you will find out what foods to buy and what not to buy. The practicalities of how to construct some lovely meals from raw ingredients are explored and the pleasures of the table and the joy of sharing food are celebrated. Beating diabetes starts in the kitchen. This is followed by an introduction to the surprisingly painless world of Fasting; mainly short intermittent fasting and restricted eating. If low-carb straightens out the chemistry, fasting can turbo-charge it to another level. The role of (modest) exercise is also presented.

The third section is short. It looks at things that may help ease change into our busy lives and what to do when we fall back or relapse.

The fourth section is a data bank of tables and other information that might be enable you to personalise your own route to effective low-carb dining. How much carb is in an alcohol drink? Which oils should I be cooking with (and why)? Were all nuts created equal? What about diabetes medicines? And much, much more.

The range of successful diets out there is vast. It seems that every diet, no matter how weird or wonderful, even the Official low-fat/low-cal ones, works for someone. Conversely, it also seems true that no single diet works for everyone. This is to be expected as biology is always diverse and there are always exceptions. The way described here works for me and, over the years, has worked for many of my patients too. You are welcome to consider it if you wish but do touch base with your healthcare professional first. Although I call it *Beating Diabetes*, a cure can never be guaranteed. Doing everything right won't work for everyone. That is just an awkward fact of life. If you have any medical conditions, or even more important, if you are on any medication, it is essential to discuss any proposed dietary change with your medical advisor before you attempt any dietary change. Unfortunately, low-carb/healthy-fat diets are likely to be viewed as cranky by many health professionals. Many of them are not (yet) aware of the benefits, nor the serious problems being caused by the Official diet advice they recommend. Be prepared.

Notes:

1. https://www.goodreads.com/quotes/66210-status-quo-you-know-is-latin-for-the-mess-we-re
2. HbA1c refers to a long-term measure of blood glucose levels. To find out more visit https://www.diabetes.org.uk/guide-to-diabetes/managing-your-diabetes/hba1c
3. Sarah Hallberg's inspiring TEDx talk 'Reversing diabetes starts with ignoring the guidelines' has inspired many. It can be viewed at: https://www.youtube.com/watch?v=da1vvigy5tQ
4. This quotation from Dr Robert Lustig can be found in an article published in the Los Angeles Times entitled 'Insulin is the bad guy' at http://articles.latimes.com/2012/jun/28/news/la-heb-calories-robert-lustig-20120628
5. Dr Jason Fung wrote 'Dr Benjamin Spock in his 1946 classic *Baby and Child Care*: 'The amount of plain starchy foods (cereals, breads, potatoes) taken is what determines…how much (weight) they gain or lose' '. https://thenoakesfoundation.org/news/blog/profs-words-what-caused-the-obesity-epidemic-expanded-foreword-to-dr-jason-fungs-new-book-the-obesity-code
6. Newspeak, a neologism coined by George Orwell and used in his novel 1984. It has been defined as 'The deliberate replacement of one set of words in the language for another.' http://www.openculture.com/2017/01/george-orwell-explains-how-newspeak-works.html.
7. A New Concept in the Treatment of Obesity. Gordon ES et al. JAMA. 1963;186(1):50-60. doi:10.1001/jama.1963.63710010013014
8. Diabesity. A word mashing up diabetes and obesity. First coined by Dr Robert Atkins.

Chapter 2 – How to get Type-2 Diabetes
How did I get it?
Why did I get it?
What can I do about it?

Getting your head around what diabetes is, what causes it and why it has happened to you will help enormously when you come to decide what you might want to do about it. Some, or even much of this is likely to be news to most of you. So, please, hang on in there. I will do my best to get all this straightened out as painlessly as possible.

Anyone who eats carbs (and we will remind ourselves exactly what they are very soon) will get a blood sugar rise and, as night follows day, anyone who gets a blood sugar rise must mount an insulin response if they are to bring their sugar level down to normal. This is indisputable. That is insulin's job. Insulin is the body's sugar controlling and energy-storage maestro and, as far as your body is concerned, glucose is a vital form of energy (Figure 2.1). It is not the only energy source, fat is an energy source too. More about fat later.

In technical terms, Type-2 Diabetes is a 'carbohydrate intolerance' disorder. This nugget of jargon simply means that you are no longer as good as you used to be at coping with the sorts of foods that push up blood sugar levels – carbs, in other words. So now, when you eat carbs, it takes longer to clear away the sugar surge that inevitably follows. In fact, as diabetes progresses, you may become unable to clear it all away, but why? What has changed?

Although insulin isn't clearing that blood sugar away anymore, weirdly it may not because you don't have enough of the stuff. Actually, early on in Type-2 Diabetes, you will have way too much insulin whooshing around. The problem is that the cells in your body that insulin links up with have started to ignore it. They have turned a deaf ear to it and the only way to make them listen is to shout louder. It does this by pushing the insulin response up. You are carb-intolerant because your body cells are insulin-deaf. The key no longer opens the door. This is insulin resistance and it is *the* underlying problem in Type-2 Diabetes (Figure 2.2).

So, let us dive into how the body really works and what actually happens when it starts to go wrong in Type-2 Diabetes. *Beating Diabetes* majors on what I call the Big-6 carbs and how they drive many of us into being overweight and diabetic. The big six are bread, pasta, pizza, rice, potatoes and sugar. More about them later. Just to say at this point that these starchy and sugary foods are the ones that commonly flood our bodies with glucose. Why? Because, chemically speaking, glucose is mostly what they are made of.

Quick apology; some of the language here is necessarily a little technical. Please bear with me. One of the great things about using the correct nomenclature is its precision. If it seems complex, just take it slowly, read it through a couple of times or even phone a friend.

The section that follows sets out clearly and precisely what diabetes is. The one that follows is a fictional timeline of the descent through the various circles of metabolic mayhem into the pit that is end-stage diabetes. Many of you with diabetes will recognise this story only too well. Your doctors and nurses most certainly will. The chapter rounds off with some essays on why you, in particular, may have developed diabetes, something about the complications of diabetes and asks (not just rhetorically) 'is diabetes a forever diagnosis?' Quick answer – not necessarily. I finish with some words about obesity.

What is diabetes?

Confusingly, there are a number of conditions that share the same name, diabetes. The two major forms are Type-1 Diabetes Mellitus and Type-2 Diabetes Mellitus. From now on when I use the word 'diabetes' I generally mean Type-2 Diabetes Mellitus. Mellitus, by the way, is a word derived from Latin and simply means honey. When diabetes was first described with its characteristically sugary urine, the only sweet thing people were familiar with was honey. Sugar as we know it was, back then, a rare, exotic and fantastically expensive commodity. Anyway, although

Types 1 and 2 may have very similar names, they are in fact totally different conditions.

Basically, in Type-1, the insulin-making cells in the pancreas gland stop working. There are a number of possible causes but the end result is that insulin no longer gets produced within the body. Type-1 is an insulin deficiency state. Typically, Type-1 develops quite suddenly and dramatically in children and teenagers; hence its now less-fashionable name, Juvenile Onset Diabetes. That name is not only unfashionable but also inaccurate. Maybe one in ten adults who develop diabetes appears to have a variant of Type-1 diabetes. One is called LADA (Latent Autoimmune Diabetes of Adults). Another, MODY (Maturity Onset Diabetes of the Young), typically affects younger adults and often runs in families. LADA tends to get labelled as Type-2 initially, which it is not. Only when the usual medicines fail to control the problem adequately might LADA or MODY be suspected. Type-1 diabetes in children usually causes weight loss, thirst and excessive urine production. It can progress quickly and cause coma and even death. Type-1 is an insulin deficiency problem and the treatment is, not surprisingly, insulin injections. For them insulin is a form of hormone replacement therapy

Before the development of insulin replacement therapy, Type-1 was almost always fatal. The only effective treatment back then was to cut out all the food items that caused blood sugar levels to rise; all the naturally sugary and starchy foods, in other words. This worked quite well as long as the person stuck to it rigidly, which is not an easy thing to do, particularly with children. These days with modern insulin injection therapy, people with Type-1 can lead pretty normal lives. Today, people with Type-1 who choose to cut down their sugar and starch consumption usually find that they need to inject less insulin. This is because the whole point of insulin injections is to control the blood sugar rises that follow eating so, the less sugary and starchy food, the fewer the blood sugar rises and less insulin needed. Insulin manufacturers are not likely to tell you this but most people with Type-1 will know it all too well. They prefer to advise you to give enough insulin to cover your food rather than modify your food to reduce your insulin requirement. I digress. Actually, people with Type-1 can also get Type-2 on top of it. It's called double diabetes, or Type-1.5 diabetes. Check the glossary for a little more detail.

In Type-2 Diabetes, the problem is precisely the opposite. In Type-2, there is initially far too much insulin. Unlike Type-1, Type-2 typically develops silently over a period of years or even decades before it starts to reveal itself. Genetic factors are involved to a certain extent. Some people and even some entire ethnic groups, are genetically more prone to developing diabetes than others. The big cause, dwarfing everything else, is diet. One commentator summed up the 'nature versus nurture' thing very nicely: 'your genes may be the gun but it's the environment that pulls the trigger'. You may have a hidden talent for getting Type-2 but it will probably not happen unless you reveal that talent by eating too much of the wrong stuff and eating it for too long. Of course, the genetic dice can also roll in your favour. You may be naturally quite resistant to developing Type-2 and able to feast on sugary and starchy foods with impunity. Lucky old you but, for most of us, a sugary and starchy diet is *the* cause of Type-2. This book is all about how diets can be mended to prevent diabetes getting worse, to reverse it and perhaps even reverse it completely. Yes, diabetes is potentially reversible. For a good many it can in effect be cured (permanently reversed that is). By the way, those same sugary and starchy carb foods are the main drivers of overweight and obesity too.

What is so bad about Type-2? Well, unlike Type-1, which is a simple deficiency disorder for which the remedy is insulin replacement injections, Type-2 is a disorder of insulin resistance and, early on, insulin excess. Insulin is the hormone of energy storage and insulin excess will promote fat accumulation and weight gain. Insulin also blocks fat release; insulin prevents weight loss. As Type-2 progresses, rising blood sugar levels can lead to internal damage.

Type-2 is essentially a chemical disorder that damages blood vessels. It can damage large blood vessels, causing heart attacks, stroke and circulation problems in the legs (which can cause gangrene and may require amputation). It can damage small blood vessels too, particularly in the eye, the kidney and around nerve fibres. The results of these are vision loss and blindness, kidney failure and numbness and tingling in the hands and particularly the feet. Type-2 is the number one reason people need kidney dialysis in the UK today. Actually, the line between Types 1 and 2 can sometimes become blurred. Bottom line: full blown Type-2, however you get it, can cause serious damage. It shortens lives and blights them with ill health.

Here's the thing. Type-2 Diabetes Mellitus is an almost totally preventable, avoidable and, early on, for some a potentially curable condition. The problem is our health services are not set up to prevent it and certainly not to cure it. Instead they have become fantastically skilled at treating it. Imagine Type-2 like an overflowing bath. Your diabetes-specialist doctors and nurses choose to use fancy syphons and are busy installing high tech extra plugholes. In other words, their approach is to bring the bath water levels down as quickly as possible. They want to empty that sugary bath as rapidly and efficiently as they can. To do this, they use the only thing they have in their toolkit - drugs. Why, I wonder, does no one do the most simple and obvious thing: just turn off the tap? Just stop pouring in the sugar. I believe that there are three reasons for this.

- Firstly, the Official diet advice given to people with Type-2 Diabetes is high-carb, which often makes things worse. It keeps tossing sugary and starchy fuel on to the flames of diabetes but fails to appreciate the link. Our doctors and nurses diligently adhere to these carb-heavy guidelines; they are pretty much obliged to. If, or when, Official dietary advice fails to reverse their diabetes, they are then obliged to prescribe drugs to counteract the effects of the very diet they promote. The aim of modern diabetes management is to slow down progression of the condition using medication, not reverse it. This is sad.

- Secondly, because their Official high-carb diet advice is almost always doomed to fail, our medics and nurses have lost confidence in the power of *any* diet or lifestyle change to heal. This is mad.

- Thirdly, to the exclusion of pretty much everything else today, the treatment of diabetes is dominated by the use of drugs. Diabetes treatments now consume around 15% of the total UK NHS budget. Diabetes is a pharmaceutical goldmine and 'Big Pharma' funds much of the medical world's influential opinion leaders and their major academic departments. Their adverts fund our medical journals. Along with the big food and drink corporations, they also fund many of the learned influential committees. They even fund national charities and support groups. Just about everyone with any power or any influence in the world of diabetes, directly or indirectly, is beholden and has a relationship with them in some way or another, whether they know it or not. At the same time, the major drug and food manufacturers keep a very firm grip on the medical world's funding streams. Big Pharma (drugs) and Big Farma (agribusiness) have no interest in preventing or curing diabetes. That isn't their job. Nor do they have the slightest interest in funding research into diet and lifestyle interventions. That isn't their job either. Their job is to sell products. For them, Type-2 Diabetes is the golden goose that just keeps on laying. Follow the money.

How to get Type-2 Diabetes Mellitus

Imagine for a moment that you really wanted to get Type-2 Diabetes Mellitus, how would you go about it? Here are the steps that typically lead from a normal healthy body chemistry through to end-stage Type-2 Diabetes. As with all things medical, there are always exceptions to the rule, but the sequence described here is what commonly happens across the world today.

1. First, choose a diet that has a good amount of sugary, starchy and processed foods. These might include bread, potato, rice, pasta, pizza and sugary drinks (the Big-6). Typically, as a young adult doing this, you will not be overweight; your blood sugar levels will be normal. Your insulin levels may be up a bit but no one ever measures them. You look good, feel great and you are as fit as a flea. You are like a calm little duck floating on a tranquil pond but, unseen, a current has developed. You have just started to paddle a little more quickly below the waterline. You are being obliged, in other words, to make a little more insulin than is desirable, to cope with your high-carb diet. You won't know this. Your doctor won't know it either and typically neither of you would be interested in changing anything anyway. Why would you? Everything is fine and dandy, isn't it?

2. Time goes by. You're in your early thirties. After another decade of carbs, your body is getting a bit fed up with all that insulin sloshing around. So, it has started becoming a bit deaf to it. You are becoming resistant to your own insulin, in other words. Not surprisingly it is called *insulin resistance*. Your body responds by making a little more insulin. That is the only way it knows to get your sugar levels back down to normal; basically, it is just shouting louder. Now all that excess insulin has started to subtly dominate your body's chemistry. You start to gain weight. Fat appears around the waist and inside the abdomen too but, apart from 'filling out' a bit, you still feel just fine. Your blood sugar levels are still in the normal range. Even with all that the extra insulin, you are coping but the current is getting stronger; that little duck has now started paddling harder, much harder. Insulin resistance, by the way, is Route-1 to getting something else; something called the Metabolic Syndrome (it's in the glossary).

3. You are now into your forties now and that 'filling out' has developed into a definite paunch; you've got a spare tyre. You may still feel fine, but blood tests would now tell you otherwise, if they were done. Your fasting

blood sugar level has risen a bit and it takes longer to clear sugar out of the bloodstream after a meal than before. Your doctor could identify these changes with fasting glucose and glucose tolerance blood tests. You would also find that your blood insulin levels were up too, if they were ever measured. The other test that might show you are approaching diabetes is the HbA1c test. This measures how much of the red stuff in your blood cells (haemoglobin) has become chemically affected by sugar (glycosylated). Red cells hang around in circulation for around three months, so the amount of glycosylated haemoglobin reflects the amount of sugar that has been around in your bloodstream during that time; more sugar, more glycosylation. It gives a fuller longer-term picture, rather than just a one-off blood-sugar snapshot, of what has been going on. Anyway, whether you know it or not, you have crossed an arbitrary line, stepped over an invisible threshold; you now have pre-diabetes. Sooner or later, most people with this will progress to Type-2 Diabetes (unless of course they turn off that metaphorical tap). That little duck is being swept downstream.

4. You are now in your fifties and at last you got that health check and those blood tests have been done and, guess what? There is a problem; it's been discovered that you now have diabetes. You still feel fine but you are fatter. Although most of those who have drifted downstream into diabetes feel good, a few will already have had some of the complications of diabetes, maybe before they even knew; problems like heart attacks, kidney or eye problems. We are all different. We all have our own unique story. The number of possible variations on the theme is huge. Anyway either your fasting glucose, your glucose tolerance or your HbA1c now says you have crossed a second invisible and arbitrary threshold. It's official, you have Type-2-Diabetes Mellitus. Congratulations and welcome to the club. At this point, your doctor and practice nurses swing into action. It is one of the things they are paid to do. It is their job and they will do it

diligently. They may well give you more of the same diet advice that got you diabetic in the first place. They will stress the joys of cutting calories to lose some weight, which will almost certainly fail. They will recommend exercise to help burn those calories, which will also almost certainly fail. I say 'almost certainly' because any intervention will work for someone. Anyway, sooner or later (usually sooner), the doctor's drug formulary book comes out of the drawer and the guidelines of learned national committees will be consulted. You suddenly find yourself on a handful of drugs each day; typically Metformin, a statin, something to bring your blood pressure down and of course some aspirin. Still no turning off the dietary tap; just drugs. You will also be told that diabetes is incurable, though if you are a very good patient (for that is what you now are) and compliant (do what you're told), you may get a remission, for a while. The expectation is that over time, your condition will progress. You will climb up a ladder (or should that be down?) of ever more potent and ever more expensive drugs, with ever more potential for side effects. Poor little duckling is in choppy waters.

5. Okay, you have now had diabetes for a few years. Your weight has stubbornly stayed put. Your medication has been increased several times. You are never away from the doctor's. You are now on first name terms with your practice nurse. Unfortunately, you may even have developed some of the complications of the diabetes but now, despite everything, your sugar levels have gone up alarmingly. Oddly, end-stage Type-2 Diabetes mimics what happens in Type-1. Those insulin-producing cells, which for decades have been pumping the stuff out like mad, get exhausted and then they fail. The current is now overwhelming. The duck's legs have finally fallen off and it is hopelessly hurtling downstream towards Niagara Falls, without a barrel. Your insulin levels have dropped. Your sugar levels have risen even higher and now your doctor says you need to start insulin injection therapy.

So, what is the answer? How can the tap be turned off and your sugar-insulin combo be restored to normal? Well, in a nutshell, you could simply do what a frustrated and overweight English undertaker called William Banting did nearly two hundred years ago; you should *avoid starch and the saccharine*[1]. In other words, cut right down on starchy foods and sugary foods and drinks. Both push glucose into the bloodstream. That metaphorical bathtub of ours is awash with sugar and the tap just keeps on pouring more in. Unless that tap is turned off, or at least turned down a lot, the bath will keep on overflowing. So now you know. That's how to get Type-2 Diabetes Mellitus.

Post script: adolescent Type-2 Diabetes Mellitus

The sequence just described is a story typical of many of those who get diabetes. However, another scenario has started to emerge in recent years and that is teenagers with Type-2 Diabetes. When dietary advice flipped in the 1980s into demonising fat and promoting carbs, the twin epidemics of diabetes and obesity (*diabesity*) took off. Two generations later we now just assume that chomping and guzzling carbs all through the day and into the night is just fine and dandy. After all, what could be better than cereals and fruit juice for breakfast and a round or two of toast before bed?

Coincidentally, during this time, as a nation we have lost much of our home cooking lore. Cooking for many is now the frustrating 20-second wait for a microwave oven to go *ping!* The preparation of wholesome meals from raw ingredients is no longer commonplace. Increasingly we have come to rely on packaged foods and takeaways. We have in effect contracted out cooking to the food industry. The consequence is that our pre-school children are fatter than they have ever been before.

In the 1960s, when I was a lad, there was just one fat boy in my whole primary school. Now, in the UK on Day-1 when 4½-year olds start infant school, there will be an average of six or seven overweight or obese children in every class of 30 children. This rises to ten or more, one third of the class, by the time they move up to secondary school. The result? Type-2 Diabetes is now being seen in teenagers who are no doubt destined to develop some of the complications of disease in early adult life, perhaps even in their twenties. Theirs is the generation that may well be outlived by their parents and perhaps even their grandparents. The effects of this disaster look like they are going to fall disproportionately on the children of less affluent and less advantaged homes. They, it seems, are also the most vulnerable to the merciless targeting by processed food, soda drinks and confectionery manufacturers. They, it seems, are more likely to eat cheap high-carb processed foods, often made even cheaper with discounted and special-offer foods, which again are almost always high-carb. They are more likely to consume high-sugar fizzy drinks and sodas. Do you think all this is an exaggeration? Well, go and check the records for dental extractions in children in your locality, a sure sign of a sugar epidemic and think again.

What is being done about it? Short answer – nothing much apart from hand-wringing in high places. Parents are confused. Our school services have no remit to sort it out. The government doesn't appear to get it and the health services have no effective answers either (although they are trying). Oh and the UK's expert body, Public Health England, has produced an App. Big deal. Meanwhile diabetes drug manufacturers and the fast-food, sugary drinks and confectionery industries keep on collecting those golden eggs. Ker-ching! After all, it isn't their problem either, is it?

Stop Press: Just as I finished writing that last paragraph, three news items popped up in just one day. The first was a statement from the UK Parliament's Health Select Committee. They published a document called *Childhood Obesity: a plan for action*. In it they recommend a policy change regarding sugar. A levy was one suggestion and a ban on the advertising of junk food to children was another. The aim was a 20% reduction in childhood sugar consumption by 2020. The government however, with one arm round the drinks industry's shoulders and the other hand being firmly sat upon, announced, *'We welcome the committee's recognition of the progress we have made in this area, delivering the most ambitious plan on childhood obesity in the world.'* Sir Humphrey, it seems, is alive and well[2].

One medically qualified Committee MP was quoted as saying "Vague statements about seeing how the current plan turns out are inadequate to the seriousness and urgency of this major public health challenge"[3]. Another complained, "We are extremely disappointed that the government has rejected a number of our recommendations. These omissions mean that the current plan misses important opportunities to tackle childhood obesity." Public Health England, not surprisingly, lined up right behind the government with their own new guidelines. Their press release said, 'The PHE guidelines are based on more than six months of meetings with the food industry and public health NGOs (Non-Governmental Organisations). More than 40 meetings were held with food suppliers, manufacturers, retailers and the eating out of home sector, representing fast food, coffee shops, family restaurants, entertainment venues and pub chains'[4]. Now, does that supping with the devil fill you with confidence?

Later that very same day, a senior doctor from PHE came on the radio, announcing that diabetes was in fact a 'walking deficiency' disorder. He had previously described sitting as the new smoking. Speaking on the same programme was yet another doctor, who correctly described Type-2 as a carbohydrate intolerance disorder with associated insulin resistance but the eminent professor was not giving any ground[5]. Diabetes, in his view, was due to sedentary office work and insufficient physical activity, in short, sloth. The role of physical activity, according to the *Beating Diabetes* approach, will be covered later in a relatively short chapter.

This all illustrates why *Beating Diabetes* has been written. National food and drink initiatives are all about politics.

Citizen's health weighs in a very distant second place; an also ran, and government agencies like PHE are obliged to line up behind their political masters. So I have to say that if you do not take responsibility for your own health and that of your family and friends, do not expect the administration to do it for you. While they churn out paper and bleat about voluntary industry change, the nation's health continues to deteriorate. In the US, Dr Robert Lustig has calculated that the total combined annual profits of the drugs and food industry combined are significantly less than the health care costs for the diseases the processed-food industries are causing. On that rather depressing note, let us swiftly move on.

Actually, not long after the parliamentary exchanges reported above, an all-parliamentary group meeting was held to discuss better ways of reversing diabetes. The session was chaired by the then MP for Leicester South, who has diabetes himself and also has some strong views on the role of sugar in society[6]. It took submissions from a variety of witnesses. In the document that followed were some amazing statements. For example, 'Type-2 Diabetes has been regarded as irreversible, steadily progressive and lifelong. Not anymore!' and 'Type-2 remission is… attainable' and 'In the UK, no one with Type-2 Diabetes should be told they have [an inevitably] progressive disease' and from a practice nurse who advises a low-carb approach 'my patients tell me I have given them hope!'[7].

Just how did I get to be diabetic?

I guess by now you probably don't need me to tell you. You can probably see who is suspect number one in having caused your diabetes. Diabetes is, for many of us, the natural human response to a high-carb diet. One eminent US doctor suggests we rename the condition *Processed Food Disease*. It seems we are all now citizens of Planet Diabetes. Of course, there are always going to be people whose metabolism will be immune to the onslaughts of the carb-insulin combo. Lucky old them but they are the exception. Most of us to a lesser or greater extent have chemical difficulties coping with our modern all-day carbohydrate lifestyle. I mentioned earlier the Big-6 carbs; bread, pizza, pasta, rice, potatoes and sugar. The first five are starchy foods that liberate glucose when eaten and they liberate it very quickly, within minutes, in fact. You could call them pre-sugar foods because sugar is what they are made of and sugar is what our body gets during digestion. For example, there is toast (sugar), porridge (sugar), spaghetti (sugar), tacos and enchiladas (sugar), baked potato (sugar), wholegrain/wholemeal bread even (sugar). Need I go on?

So, if (bad luck) you are very sensitive to sugary and starchy foods and are diabetic or pre-diabetic, or overweight, there are two paths you can go by (sic Led Zeppelin's Stairway to Heaven). You need to choose. You can enter through a wide gate and follow the path of full-frontal medical management and drug treatment. The range of drugs out there is comprehensive and your nurses and medics are highly skilled at managing diabetes. Their aim is to slow disease progression down and to try and reduce your risk of getting any of its horrid complications. It is a form of managed retreat. It is a policy of acquiescence. It is a strategy designed to slow down the inevitable, in other words. On the other hand, you could just slip quietly through the narrow gate on to the low-carb path and head towards the chance of getting into remission from your diabetes. Actually there are two other proven ways to reverse diabetes; bariatric surgery and very low calorie diet intervention programmes. In reality, most people who opt for the low-carb way try to do so in concert with their medics. After all, if you plan to stop the carb-drive into diabetes in its tracks, it is absolutely essential first to talk to your doctor about your medications.

Unfortunately, the view most medics have of diabetes is that it is linked pretty much exclusively to just one thing, being overweight (Figures 2.2 & 2.3). Being pragmatic, realistic sorts of people and knowing all too well how difficult it is to lose weight, they see little point in advising a serious trial of lifestyle change. Why waste time? Much better to whack you straight on to Metformin, which will rapidly improve your laboratory results profile. Good enough? Well, your glucose and HbA1c levels will almost certainly improve, at least for a while. They will, of course, advise you to lose weight and comply with the Official dietary guidelines. However, as the Official guidance is high-carb heavy, you are likely to find the sugary driving force underlying your diabetes eventually overwhelms the 'insulin sensitising' effects of Metformin. You are going to need to take more drugs and so it goes.

So, obesity and diabetes are in most cases the result of eating starchy and sugary carbs, not eating fatty foods. Obesity and diabetes are the results of a disordered metabolism and not their cause. Let's just read that again because it is dynamite. Obesity and diabetes are the results of, the 'consequences of' in other words, a disordered metabolism and *not* their cause. What it means is that being overweight or obese does not the cause diabetes. Rather, both diabetes and obesity are the result of our officially sanctioned high-carb insulin-provoking dietary advice.

Let us use a little bit of logic. Here is a sequence of statements. They are all factual and your doctors and nurses will no doubt agree with each and every one of them.

1. Dietary carbohydrates cause blood glucose levels to rise during digestion.
2. Sugary and processed starchy foods cause blood glucose levels to rise higher than fibrous low-carbohydrate food, like those found in most vegetables.
3. A rise in blood glucose obliges the body to release insulin to bring glucose level down to normal.
4. Glucose will be taken up by cells that need to use it straight away and, if necessary, it will replenish the body's glucose stores – glycogen. After that, insulin converts all remaining glucose into fat.
5. Insulin helps drive fat out of the circulation into fat cells for storage
6. Insulin blocks the release of fat from fat cells.

7. Persistent insulin secretion (from eating too many carbs for example) can cause cells to become less sensitive to its effects (insulin resistance).
8. Insulin resistance obliges the body to secrete higher levels of the hormone to overcome the block and to keep blood glucose levels down in the normal range.
9. When insulin resistance becomes severe, the body loses its ability to control glucose levels effectively (pre-diabetes and diabetes).
10. In the long-term, high glucose levels and fat accumulation within the pancreas damage the insulin-producing cells in the pancreas, which can lead to a fall in insulin secretion. This happens late in established Type-2 Diabetes.
11. Insulin production failure is followed by even higher blood sugar levels and this requires treatment with insulin injections.

From point No. 9 and onwards, you will find your doctors and nurses becoming very interested in you, that is clinically interested. This is not a surprise. It is because these are the pre-diabetic and Type-2 diabetic stages. Even by the time you reach Point No. 11, what many consider a locked-in stage of diabetes, a low-carb diet may still help. You may be able to cut your insulin dose significantly and lose some weight but it would need to be done extremely carefully, bearing in mind the number of anti-diabetic drugs you would be on by then.

The *Beating Diabetes* approach sees things differently. It sees the whole problem as one of excessive dietary carb intake, especially the potent sugary and starchy ones. This state of affairs develops steadily over years and decades. *Beating Diabetes* contends that drastically cutting down on sugary and starchy foods can stop the process rolling on inexorably deeper into diabetes. If you don't cut the carbs, you are likely to end up treating your food choices with drugs (read that sentence again) but if you can restore a normal metabolism by cutting your carbs (as can happen in most people), then you may well be able to turn your back on disease progression. This can reduce or even stop your need for drug treatments and reverse your medically managed decline. At each and every one of the 11 points listed above, cutting carbs reduces and can potentially turn the whole process around.

This is not some fancy theory. One GP in the north of England has shown that it can really work in practice. Dr David Unwin came across the potential benefits of the low-carb approach some years ago and went on to devise a programme within his own practice for people with diabetes. He made a point of stressing the blood sugar raising potential of a number of starchy carb foods; five of the Big Six, basically. He devised something he called 'the Tea-spoon Equivalent' which gave his patients an idea of the amount of sugar locked away within many starchy foods. For example, the TSEs for typical servings of broccoli, banana and basmati rice are around $1/5^{th}$, 5½ and 10 teaspoons respectively. So, a 150g serving of rice raises your blood sugar by the same amount as swallowing around 10 teaspoons full of table sugar. You can see the TSEs of many other foods at the Public Heath Collaboration's website[8]. With this brilliantly simple approach, David and his colleagues have managed to move from being Southport's highest prescribers of diabetes drugs to its lowest. They have impressive patient data going back over several years on the benefits of a low-carb approach in both overweight and diabetic patients. Indeed, many of his patients are now enthusiastic advocates working on the programme.

What's so bad about diabetes?

- Bad luck. You have become a patient – most people who become diabetic will get stuck in the never-ending rut of being a patient. You will be given pills if you are lucky and injections and pills if you are not. You will be recalled endlessly for check-ups and monitoring and because, unbeknown to your nurses and doctors, the standard diet advice at best does nothing much (and can make things worse), you will be ever so politely ticked off on a regular basis for your failures; failure to lose weight and failure to get your HbA1c down.

- You now have a disease label – sorry about this, but you are now a person attached to a disease. You may have thought you were a person with diabetes but, as far as health professionals are concerned, you are now a diabetic, a case. Make sure you like your doctors and nurses; you are going to see a lot more of them over the next few years.

- Oh and you will have to take drugs of one sort or another – Metformin is the usual entry level medication and, like any drug that is any good, there is the potential for side effects. With Metformin, feeling sick, tummy pains and diarrhoea are not uncommon. It usually works pretty well at dampening down the insulin resistance that is driving the whole diabetic show. It does not, however, induce remission. Medication rarely reverses diabetes. It is a pharmacological coping strategy; it simply reduces the problem for a while. Metformin is an excellent medication, but if your glucose control is not good enough, there are many other drugs that can be used. There are, in fact, eight different classes of anti-diabetic drugs, plus insulin. Many people with diabetes take two or three different anti-diabetic drugs in combination (See Appendix 7).

- Finally, you are at risk of getting complications associated with diabetes. The big deal about diabetes is not particularly what your blood sugar score is. It is the underlying metabolic condition that damages blood vessels. The blood vessels that take the hit are large arteries, like those found in the brain and the heart and small arteries, like those in the eye, the kidney and surrounding nerves in your limbs. The medical jargon for these complications is macro-vascular and micro-vascular damage. To protect your large arteries, you may well be given cholesterol-lowering drugs (commonly a statin), plus medication to control blood pressure and an aspirin. These reduce the chances of micro-vascular damage too. All these drugs and their effects need to be monitored regularly with blood and urine tests, eye check-ups and skin-prick tests for numbness. Just to throw another spanner in the works, some people will get complications of diabetes before they even know they have been diagnosed as having diabetes. The first signs of diabetes could be a problem with your sight, or chest pain, for example. Of course, as with any long-term condition, it can take a toll on mental health and wellbeing. None of this sounds very cheerful. In reality, there is life after being diagnosed with diabetes. It is just a bit different. Bottom line: if you could reverse the process and potentially even reverse the condition and perhaps be able to drop some of the drugs as well, ... why wouldn't you?

Will I always be diabetic?

There are two possible answers here and the one you get depends on who you ask.

The current medical view is – yes. Once a diabetic, always a diabetic. You may go into remission but (sorry buddy) it's temporary, because you ARE a diabetic. You have got it. So, if someone manages to turn their lifestyle around and all the blood markers of diabetes go away, it is very unlikely that their doctor will expunge the diagnosis from their medical records; because you have got diabetes, stupid. This is a circular form of logic. The diabetic label is a very sticky one.

The other view is – no. It is possible to reverse diabetes, to get your blood glucose and HbA1 levels back to normal and, if caught early enough, come off drugs too; a cure if you will. This is because diabetes is seen as a hormonal or metabolic state and not a disease entity and because metabolic (or body chemistry) states can recover, then obviously diabetes can recover too; Type-2 Diabetes is potentially reversible. Having insulin resistance potent enough to make you diabetic is amenable to dietary change. Most medics don't acknowledge it but deep down they already know this. It is well known and accepted that bariatric surgery (stomach stapling or gastric bands for example) can cure diabetes, even Type-2s on insulin. Yet many still consider encouraging diet change to be ineffective. Of course, as has been said several times already, nothing works for everyone and so the low-carb approach can never be guaranteed 100% to work but what you can guarantee with a fair degree of certainty is that continuing a on high-carb diet will keep the diabetes bubbling away nicely. So, hey, I say to my patients, what have you got to lose by trying a low-carb diet? There are two other 'of courses' we need to add. Firstly, if you have already been damaged by the diabetes, lost some vision or had a heart attack, for example, changing your diet won't cure that. That clock cannot be turned back. Diet-change will, however, offer some protection against further trouble. The second 'of course' is that for those people with Type-2 Diabetes who are on diabetes drugs or insulin injection therapy, any dietary and fasting changes must be made very carefully indeed and with close expert medical advice. Some anti-diabetic drugs must be taken with food, sometimes carb-food in particular. If you don't take them with a meal, they could produce a drop in your blood glucose levels and cause a hypo (hypoglycaemic attack). Hypos can be very dangerous. See Appendix 7 for information about diabetes drugs.

A word or two about obesity

Everyone agrees overweight and obesity rates are on the rise. The Official advice given by most health professionals to help lose weight is to cut calories, eat plenty of starchy carbs and take a little more exercise. None of these usually makes much of a dent in the underlying problem driving everything headlong towards the cliff; excessive insulin levels. In fact, following Official dietary advice often does the opposite. It keeps the whole sugar-insulin-combo show rolling on and, just to make calorie-controlled dieting even more useless, it has a nasty habit of slowing down the body chemistry; it reduces the body's metabolic rate, in other words. When the body slows down to cope with food restriction, it goes into frugal-mode; it starts to make do with fewer calories. Frustratingly, when those goalposts move, weight loss gets even tougher. The harder you cut back, the harder the body slows up its calorie burning.

So, what happens? The overweight beat themselves up and their health professionals do a lot of tut-tutting. Most people I know who have successfully lost significant amounts of weight have not done so with the help of their doctor or nurse (unless they have had a gastric band operation for example). Most have either joined a commercial slimming club or found out for themselves what their health professionals were not telling them; that it's the carb-insulin combo that generally makes you fat and it's the carb-insulin combo that keeps you fat.

Distinguishing between causation and association is crucial in trying to get to the truth but all too often medics and scientists just need to get their papers published. Combine this with statistically naïve journalism and, before you know it, associations get conflated deviously into what sounds like causation; fake news if you will. If you would like a nice association to chew on, how about this. The obesity and diabetes epidemics began in the United States and UK in the 1980s and ever since they have been building like a tsunami, ever higher, year upon year. The diabesity epidemic cannot be genetic; it has happened way too quickly for that to be the explanation. It has to be environmental; nurture not nature, in other words. Anyway, in February 1977, US Senator George McGovern's Senate Committee fired the starting gun for the low-fat high-carb diet revolution. They did this by profoundly changing the food advice given to Americans, based on their belief in the diet-heart hypothesis (See the glossary entry). These two things, a change in food advice and the start of the epidemic, are very neatly associated in time. If you ask me, I would say that McGovern's low-fat high-carb eating revolution looks pretty causative and, if you would like to see an impressive illustration of the scale of the problem, why not visit the Centre for Disease Control and Prevention website and scroll through their PowerPoint slides. Better make sure you are sitting down first[9].

And what can I do about it?

The long answer to the question, I might tell my patients, is… read the rest of the book. This is the best way to nail all the details, all the ins and outs and to avoid pitfalls. In doing so, you should be painlessly enabled and find your own way to making changes effectively. Of course, I would say that, though, wouldn't I?

If you really need to know right now, well here it is. Cut the sugary and starchy foods in what you eat, take a modest amount of exercise, miss the odd meal particularly breakfast, or have calorie-light days once in a while (that sounds so much less threatening than fasting) and no snacking. Do these things and your blood sugar levels should start dropping immediately. Your insulin levels should start dropping immediately too. This should cut your insulin resistance down within about three or four weeks. Most people who follow a low-carb approach will, over a few weeks, find their fasting glucose, glucose tolerance test and their HbA1c all improve. Oh, and your triglyceride levels should drop too. Most people will see a drop in weight and belt size as well. This will not work for everyone, because nothing ever does but it should work for most people with diabetes by correcting the underlying problem with body chemistry; insulin resistance and insulin excess.

Conclusion

Okay readers, well done. Pat yourselves on the back. Welcome to Planet Diabetes, you steered your way through some background history, from the Stone Age through the agricultural and pastoral revolutions, through agri-business and into our current diabesity pandemic. You have discovered that the Official advice out there on diabetes is an edifice built on the shifting sands of scientific error; fats don't make you fat; carbs make you fat. It's the carbs that have driven us headlong into an epidemic of diabesity. Why most of our experts refuse to acknowledge this is an enigma wrapped in a mystery. In this chapter we have also addressed some of the scientific thinking behind the low-carb approach for diabetes You have had to endure some techno-jargon but hey, no pain, no gain. Now, let us move on swiftly to the first of the *Beating Diabetes* 'how to do it' sections. Just which foods work with our body chemistry when it comes to diabetes and which foods assuredly do not? You may get a few surprises.

Figure 2.1 What happens when you eat starchy and sugary foods

Eat a sugary or starchy meal	For example: bread, pasta, pizza, rice, potato, most processed foods, most "low-fat" foods, sweetened drinks and sodas, confectionery, table sugar, and even fruit
Which produces a rise in blood glucose levels	Starchy foods rapidly liberate glucose during digestion. Sugary foods and drinks contain glucose and another sugar called fructose
Which provides immediate-use fuel for bodily functions	Like walking, talking, thinking, dreaming, breathing, creating, procreating, peeing, pooping, shivering, yawning, growing hair, or scratching your nose even
And which tops up our on-board sugar stores (muscle and liver glycogen, basically)	Glycogen is a form of starch; a concentrated chain of sugary glucose molecules. Muscles use it up during exercise. The liver uses it to keep blood glucose levels up between meals and overnight
Then... **ALL** remaining glucose is converted by insulin into **FAT** and stored	When glycogen stores are full, any glucose not needed immediately for bodily activity is converted into fat, stored in fat cells and kept there by insulin. This is obligatory. It is the glucose/insulin combination that makes you fat, and keeps you fat. It is the carb-insulin combo that drives diabetes

Figure 2.1: Of course, most real meals have some fat and protein in them too. In low-carb meals fats and proteins become more important sources of fuel. Fats do not require insulin to work.

Figure 2.2 The two pathways to Type-2 Diabetes Mellitus

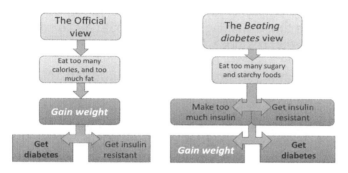

Figure 2.2 The difference between these two pathways is significant. The Official view contends that simply eating too much gets you fat and being fat causes diabetes. It demonises obesity. The low-carb view suggests otherwise. It says a carb-heavy diet *causes* insulin resistance and this then leads to both diabetes and obesity (diabesity).

Figure 2.3 The two responses to Type-2 Diabetes Mellitus

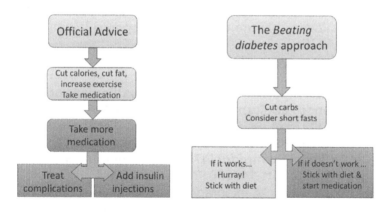

Figure 2.3 Because the Official view chose the wrong pathway to start with, it was obliged to advise the wrong response too. Official management at best just eases the brakes on the progress of diabetes – perhaps a bit. *Beating Diabetes* is a U-turn in the road, using forward and reverse gears. Low-carb dieters who do need medication will

usually need less of it than those following Official advice.

Notes:

(1) William Banting, who died nearly two hundred years ago, advised those wishing to lose weight to *avoid starch and the saccharine.* His book *Letter on Corpulence* was published in 1863. The full text can be found at **https://onlinelibrary.wiley.com/doi/pdf/10.1002/j.1550-8528.1993.tb00605.x**

(2) Sir Humphrey Appleby was a fictional civil servant in the BBC TV series Yes minister and Yes Prime minister. He was 'a master of **obfuscation** and manipulation, often making long-winded statements to confuse and fatigue the listener.' **https://en.wikipedia.org/wiki/Humphrey_Appleby**

(3) **http://www.nationalhealthexecutive.com/Health-Care-News/government-warned-to-take-robust-action-against-child-obesity-**

(4) **https://www.gov.uk/government/news/guidelines-on-reducing-sugar-in-food-published-for-industry**

(5) Leading doctor claims Type-2 diabetes is 'just down to laziness' **https://closeronline.co.uk/diet-body/health-fitness/doctor-sir-muir-gray-type-2-diabetes-walking-deficiency-syndrome/**

(6) An article about Leicester South's MP. **https://www.bbc.co.uk/news/uk-england-leicestershire-34744976**.

(7) Catherine Cassell, Practice nurse with a special interest in diabetes **http://www.parliament.wa.gov.au/parliament/commit.nsf/(Evidence+Lookup+by+Com+ID)/BF4B4A16278DE6CC4825832300252430/$file/20181008+-+T2D+SUB+10+-+Mr+David+Unwin.pdf** & **https://mailchi.mp/ddf447abb1da/reversingtype-2-diabetes-report-1472601?e=8b2ca66d84**

(8) See Dr Unwin's infographics on the 'teaspoons of sugar equivalents' of various common foods at **https://phcuk.org/sugar/**.

Part 2

We gotta get out of this place

Chapter 3 – Shop

Let food be your **medicine**[1]

In the last chapter, we discovered that the number one thing driving our diabesity epidemic over a cliff is carbohydrate food. Not all carbs though. Not fibre-rich vegetables, just the potent sugary and starchy ones but what does this mean in practice? What can the budding diabetic do about it? How can you dodge the carbs? What, in fact, shall we have for dinner?

Just to kick things off with some clarity, Table 3.1 compares the advice most Official diets give about the healthy eating with *Beating Diabetes'* very different low-carb message. I find the chemistry lesson approach a bit confusing, especially when so few foods are formed exclusively of one food chemical alone, e.g. meat, which is a mix of protein and fats both saturated and unsaturated. When I shop, I do not make a beeline for some saturated fat, nor do I sidestep the carbohydrate cabinet. No, I buy real food. Nevertheless, if you are interested, you can glance at Table 3.1 and note the significant difference between Official guidance and the low-carb approach. I have included Omega-6 fats in this table. It will become clear, in due course, why I believe that these edible food substances (sorry, cannot quite bring myself to call them foods) should be minimised too, despite their undoubted culinary qualities.

In this chapter, you will also find specific advice about a range of foods, by which I mean ingredients, ingredients being the produce that can be conjured into a meal. If you are in a hurry to know, have a look at the In-Foods/Out-Foods lists (Tables 3.2 and 3.3). These roughly divide the various types of foods into those to be preferred and those to be avoided, or at least minimised. It's a sheep and goats thing. Actually, I don't believe that any food should be absolutely considered 'Out'. Perhaps industrial trans-fats might be the exception that proves the rule. The lists are quick-glance things. Much more useful information is given in the pages that follow. So, if you really want to know exactly why fruit and the 5-a-day thing may not be so good for you if have diabetes, then sorry, you will just have to just keep on reading.

One more point before we set off for the shops; there is nothing new about the low-carb approach. Avoiding sugary and starchy foods was the norm for a century before the high-carb era was ushered in in the 1980s. Since then there have been many more advocates for low-carb dining. Robert Atkins was one, David Jenkins and the GI approach was another. More recently dietdoctor.com[2] and Professor Aseem Malhotra and Donal O'Neill's excellent *Pioppi Diet* advocates strongly for the health benefits of avoiding sugary and starchy foods.

Table 3.1 A comparison of Official Guidance and the *Beating Diabetes low-carb* approach for healthy eating for people with diabetes

Food Group	Examples	Official Guidance	*Low-carb says...*
Fat	Meat, fish, dairy, eggs, dairy, nuts, vegetable oils	Modest amounts only	Enjoy
- Saturated fat	Meat, fish, dairy, eggs, dairy, nuts	Minimise	Enjoy
- Omega-6 fats	Rapeseed, corn oil, vegetable oils, soya products, margarine	Poly-unsaturated Omega-6 heavy oils are good. Use in preference to real fats and oils	Avoid! Choose real fats and oils, preferably every time
Carbohydrates	Sugary, starchy and fibre foods	Base all meals generously on this food group	Caution! True vegetables good, other carbs not so good
- Sugar	Table sugar, sweetened sodas, honey, and any number of sugar like chemicals	Limit	Avoid, avoid, avoid!
- Sugary foods	Fruit	5-a-day good, 10-a-day better	Minimal quantities. For pleasure only, not health
- Starchy foods	Grain-based foods (e.g. bread, pizza, pasta, rice) and starchy veg' e.g. potato, beetroot	Base all meals on this food group	Avoid
- Low-carb carbs	Everything from asparagus to zucchini via broccoli and cabbage	Include regularly	Enjoy in abundance
Protein foods	Some of the above like meat, eggs, dairy, fish, plus pulses	Beans and pulses good	Beans and pulses okay in modest quantities unless you need to go very low-carb for control

Table 3.1: See **http://www.nhs.uk/Livewell/Goodfood/Pages/the-eatwell-guide.aspx** for pictorial representation and explanations on Official guidance and **https://patient.info/doctor/diabetes-diet-and-exercise** for UK NHS food advice for people with Type-2 Diabetes (including the UKs DESMOND programme – Diabetes Education and Self-management for Ongoing and Newly Diagnosed)

No, nothing is under an absolute ban. Just make sure your off-piste indulgences are modest, infrequent and, importantly, enjoyable. I say enjoyable because there is in fact no other good reason to eat anything from the Out-Foods list at all. So, if you want to eat fish and chips on the beach, make sure they are good and that you dine on them. Sit down and celebrate – no brainless scoffing on the move. We will talk about dining later. So, never commit dietary sins mindlessly. Two points must be made here; firstly, indulging in Out-Foods should be a rare treat and secondly, you must be very sure it is worth it. There is absolutely no point being naughty if it is not very nice and, because those sugary and starchy Out-Foods will wash sugar into your bloodstream, why not consider slowing down the *insulin-turns-sugar-into-fat* conveyor belt by programming in some strategic exercise? That way some of the sugar will be diverted into your muscles. For example, precede that fish and chip supper with a swim or brisk half-hour walk. Or perhaps follow the meal with another power walk, or do both. Exercise will burn off some of the sugar and perhaps some of your muscle glycogen too which will then have to be replenished from your blood sugar. More about exercise later.

Something you may also notice is that almost all the foods discussed in this chapter are ingredients. They are raw materials that can, through culinary magic, be transformed into lovely meals. Pre-prepared, packaged and factory facsimiles of real meals are not included in this section. This is because I do not automatically consider them as real foods even if they are edible, and even if they taste good. Again, more on this and the dangers of contracting out your cooking to anonymous industrial third parties and the joys of real cooking later. Oh, and see Appendix 6 for how to navigate the minefield that is food labelling.

Before we go any further – a wee word about Oils and Fats

In the 1950s, an American scientist got it into his mind that the root of all things cardiac-evil was fat; saturated fat to be precise. He then set about doing two things with characteristic vigour. He began collecting evidence to prove he was right, and then mercilessly trashed anyone who disagreed with him. What he should have done was looked for evidence to prove he was wrong. That, weirdly is the safest scientific way to determine the truth; strange but true. And secondly, suppressing any debate on the subject said more about his domineering and controlling personality than his scientific credentials. Sadly, what he considered his great gift to humanity, the diet-heart hypothesis, proved instead to be a curse. And even though he has now been shown to be wrong, posthumously, the poisonous little thought that "fat is dangerous" has bored its way into our collective consciousness, and for many it sits there still; a piece of default but erroneous software lodged in our brains.

You see, fats do not cause heart disease at all. They never did, and had anyone bothered to look at the high-quality evidence that was already there in the literature in the 1960s, much suffering could have been avoided. But our brainy scientists and medics didn't, and nor did our politicians. Instead, food producers stepped up to the plate, did as they were told, and cut the saturated fat from as many foods as they could. Of course, all that fat had to be replaced with something, and I think by now you will know what it got replaced with. That's right; sugar and starchy flour, plus the newly developed industrial seed oils (poly-unsaturated fats), and salt. Sneaking under the low-fat radar, high-carb processed foods got in (along with the industrially produced poly-unsaturated seed oils) and they have been killing us ever since.

Are all fats good or are some less good than others? The answer to that is caveat emptor; let the buyer beware. Fats and oils fall conveniently into two groups; naturally occurring ones like olive oil, oily fish, butter and lard on the one hand, and the industrially extracted seed oils like canola, rape, soy, sunflower and a number of other 'vegetable oils' on the other. The natural ones have been around for, well forever, and the industrial seed oils for a few decades. Neither has any effect on blood sugar or insulin levels and so are not directly linked to the diabesity story. But they do differ from one another in one very significant particular: the industrial seed oils all contain a high concentration of Omega-6 fat.

Omega-3 and Omega-6 fats are vital for good health; indeed, food scientists call them essential fatty acids. They are called essential because although we need them, our bodies cannot manufacture them. We need to get them from somewhere else; in short, we need to eat them to stay healthy. Before agriculture was invented, it is estimated that the ratio between Omega-3 and Omega-6 in the diet varied between 1:1 and 1:10. However, the amount of Omega-6 fatty acids consumed in most modern diets has increased greatly (perhaps with the exception of the so-called Mediterranean diet). A ratio of 1:25 is now commonly quoted, though for some it could be closer to 1:40 or even 1:50. The concern is that an Omega-6 excess can cause inflammatory problems within the body. Inflammatory problems include things like arthritis and coronary heart disease. So, for this reason, I choose to cook and dine with "natural" fats like butter, olive oil and sometimes coconut oil. I choose these because having had "heart issues" myself, the less inflammation my poor old coronary arteries are exposed to in future the better. You see, inflammation and disordered blood clotting and tissue repair are the true causes of coronary artery disease, not cholesterol. But I digress.

Appendix 1 lists a number of fats and oils and gives figures for Omega-3s, 6s and their ratio. You can see there that the industrial seed oils are all, without exception, high Omega-6 oils in both absolute and ratio terms.

Table 3.2 The Quick-Glance In-Foods List

In-Foods	Pick your foods and ingredients mainly from this list. There are plenty to choose from.

Meat	All meat is acceptable – as long as it's not in pies or pastry, breaded or battered. Do not worry about fat but beware gravy (often made with flour or potato starch). Watch out when buying processed meats like sausage which can hide bread, rusk and even things like apple in their recipe
Fish	All seafood is acceptable – as long as it's not battered or breaded, or accompanied by portions of chips. Fish, mussels, prawns, scallops, calamari, roe are all fine. Enjoy
Dairy	Good in moderation. Enjoy cheese but not on toast or in sandwiches. Caution with yoghurt, some products hide a lot of sugar. Anything called low-fat is almost always high-sugar
Vegetables	All true vegetables are fine. Boil, bake, shred, stir-fry, steam or spiralise them; eat them raw, even. Potatoes and similar roots are exceptions
Poultry	All fowl is fair, but again not battered or breaded and not in floury sauces, nor in sandwiches or pies
Eggs	Go to work on an egg, have a day-off on an egg, but no Scotch eggs with their breaded coats on
Nuts	Nuts are fine, but avoid nuts in chocolate (or anything else)
Mushrooms	Tasty, low-carb but not in breadcrumbs or batter, please
Sauces	Beware, many hide flour or potato starch. Real mayonnaise is fine if it's the proper stuff made only with egg and olive oil. If the label says "low" or "reduced" fat, avoid it as it almost always means it has added sugars and starch

Plus, a couple of almost In-Foods...

Beans and pulses	Beans and lentils are fine in small quantities. But read the label first. Some are sweetened with sugar or thickened with flour. Some call pulses "carbs masquerading as protein". On average they come in around 15-20% carb, but they vary quite a lot. Read the food information label or check in a carb-counter book
Berries	A small handful, two or three times a week is fine. Eat them whole. No juicing
Wine	...is fine in moderation and as long as it's dry, not sweet. Champagne, they say, of all the wines, has the lowest effect on blood sugar. Spirits have no direct effect on blood sugar at all, but because of their potency should be enjoyed only occasionally
Sweeteners	Saccharin, aspartame etc. Hmm, I'm not 100% sure here. For me, the jury is out. Any industrially produced edible substance is suspect, even if it's zero-cal. Recent evidence suggesting they boost insulin secretion is a significant worry for me

Table 3.3 The Quick-Glance Out-Foods List

Out-Foods	Out-Foods and ingredients are ones that cause blood sugar levels to rise rapidly and stay up for a long time. They oblige the body to pump out extra insulin. And too much insulin is a real problem in diabetes. So, minimise your consumption of the foods listed below.
Bread...	Flour is starch, a carb made from chains of glucose. If you must have it, then eat it. But, eat only small portions; an occasional treat. If you must have it frequently, then stop reading now and give this book to someone else
...and other flour products	Sorry, biscuits, cakes, crispy snacks, pastries, bagels, croutons...it's all starch and that means it is a high-energy carb. Avoid
Rice	That S-word again. Another starchy grain. Small portions, occasional servings. If you must have rice frequently...stop reading now
Potatoes and similar roots	"Potato Pete" boasted in wartime Britain "I'm an energy food." That energy is starch (glucose chains). I like chips but have then only two or three times a year – an occasional treat, part of a feast rather than one of my staples
Beer	...or liquid bread. Unlike wine, beers and lagers are made from malted barley, and malt (or maltose to give it its proper name) is a sugar. I enjoy a pint myself, but it's an occasional treat and not a regular thing now
Sugar	The ultimate nutrition-free edible product. It's hidden in almost every processed food you buy now, even bran flakes and muesli. Read food labels, hunt it down and assiduously avoid! And look out for weasel ways of sneaking sugars into foods without mentioning them directly on the label – dextrose, fructose, corn syrup, honey to name but four. Sugar is hidden in things like tomato ketchup, non-diet cola drinks and many cocktails, sausages, and, until recently, sometimes even toothpaste. And it is, of course, the main ingredient in confectionery. If the product says it has no added sugar, it may mean there is plenty in it naturally (intrinsic sugar – see glossary). Beware. Table sugar (sucrose) is half fructose, half glucose. Fructose in anything other than small amounts is a real health hazard. A clear and present danger. Avoid!
Don't panic	Actually, there are no banned foods with the *Beating Diabetes* approach. Just make sure that any Out-Foods you eat feature infrequently and in small portions...and are worth it (i.e. make sure you enjoy them)

Plus, an almost Out-Food...

Fruit	Ignore the propaganda. Fruit is high-fructose tree candy. Fruit is not a health food. Eat it if you enjoy it, but eat it whole and eat it fresh. Dried fruit is a concentrated carb food-bomb. So...no smoothies, no fruit juices, no fruit in syrup or sprinkling it with sugar either. Aim for a maximum of one small portion per day if you must have it. Only eat fruit for pleasure, not health

Meat, Poultry and Fish

We humans are by nature omnivorous, well suited to eating a range of both animal and plant foods. Indeed, the range of foods humans do not just survive on but thrive on is diverse in the extreme. Of course, these days it is even possible to thrive without meat. Yes, thanks to centuries of plant husbandry, improvement and development (soft genetic modification, if you will), strict vegetarianism is no longer a death sentence.

With the *Beating Diabetes* approach, no meats, poultry or fish are excluded, though you must be eagle-eyed with processed forms like sausages. I suppose we could get a little picky about farmed salmon and the abomination that is corn-fed beef. Both disturb the Omega-3/6 balance of the produce, not to mention the degraded lives exclusively corn-fed cattle are subjected to. Do you see great herds of wildebeest migrating across the African savannah in search of corn? No. They eat grass, as do all ruminants. It shouldn't be a surprise therefore, that corn-fed beef is nutritionally inferior to the natural grass-fed variety.

So, all flesh is fair as long as it is not tainted with carbohydrate. No pastry jackets or breaded coatings; no crusty pies, no using them to fill wraps or sandwiches, open or otherwise and no dousing them in floury or potato-thickened sauces, or drizzling them with sugary dressings and marinades. If you buy a BBQ sauce, read the label very carefully. Most are BBQ-smoke flavoured sugary syrups.

Just be aware that processed meats can quietly sneak the carbs in too. That meaty sausage might have a flour or rusk filler. They may also have flavoursome ingredients like Bramley apple which can bump the sugar-hit up to around two teaspoons per banger. Another highish-carb flavoured sausage incorporates caramelised onion. The clue here is in the name: caramelised. The same can be said of some meat pâtés and pastes. If in doubt, check the food label; no, not the diabolical multi-coloured advertising information graphics on the front, but the full table of information, usually sneaked in somewhere out of the buyer's line of sight in much smaller print. The renowned food journalist and writer Michael Pollan once said something like 'never eat a food that makes a health claim'. If a food product says it is low in sugar, as for example did some sausages I bought recently, they may well have a very high starchy carb content and, as far as the body is concerned, starchy carbs are in fact... yes... sugar. The sneaking in of misleading and partial truths on packaging is a dark art and our shops and supermarkets are awash with it. Perhaps you should just avoid food that comes in packages?

Milk, Dairy and Eggs

Milk has always been in our diets, but only for infants. The only truly natural dairy product is mother's breast milk. What we love and enjoy now is in fact baby food for cows, goats or sheep. Animal milk only entered the human food chain when wild cattle, sheep and goats were first domesticated 7-8,000 years ago. Since then, careful breeding and cross-breeding have provided us with a range of veritable milk-producing machines. They are called dairy herds. Milk does, of course, contain sugar, a very special one called lactose. Lactose is a double sugar, half glucose half galactose. It needs an enzyme in the bowel called lactase to split it into its simple single sugar constituents before it can be absorbed. If you do not split it yourself during digestion, bugs in your lower bowel will do it for you. The result – bloating and gassy diarrhoea. The lactase enzyme is in short supply in some people of Afro-Caribbean and East Asian ancestry. If they drink milk, they may well find that they get lactose intolerance symptoms.

When milk is turned into cheese, most of the lactose is skimmed off with the watery whey. The result is that cheese, particularly hard cheeses like cheddar and parmesan, have far less lactose sugar than in whole milk. Soft cheeses like feta may have a higher lactose carb content. They vary. Cheeses are generally very low-carb foods. Caution: some processed cheeses can have sugars added to prolong their shelf life and prevent them going off.

Yogurts are a bit of a halfway house between milk and cheese. Their sugar content is very variable, not least because many of them have sugars and fruit added to sweeten and flavour them. The sweeter high-carb yoghurts are likely to be promoted as low-fat. The unsweetened fruit yogurts will boast 'no added sugar'. This is technically true, but here is a hint: for fruit, read sugar. The same goes for salad dressing, by the way. Low-*anything* is almost always a smoke screen for High-*something else*. *Caveat emptor*, I say again. Read the food information box and not just the multi-coloured carefully chosen and frequently partially true bits on the front of the package. Those traffic-lights are highly selective about what they present, which can make them misleading. Remember, the blurb on the front of the packets and packages is predominately promotional in nature, partial information to persuade you to buy and consume. It is, in my view, advertising.

Anyway, milk is around 4.5% carbohydrate, which isn't much unless you drink a lot of it. The carb content of skimmed, semi-skimmed and full fat milk is similar. The water and fat contents do vary, however. Butter, cream, natural cheese and low-sugar plain yoghurts are generally low-carb and, assuming they do not upset your tummy, are fine to enjoy. Processed milk products like evaporated milk and condensed milk (50% sugar), milk fruit-shakes and chocolate milk all usually have added sugars and are to be avoided. Also to be avoided are combinations of dairy products with carb foods. Cheese sandwiches, cheese on toast, cheese on biscuits, cheesy sauces with flour, yoghurt granola bars even. It is all pretty obvious, when you think about it. See Appendix 4 for fuller technical details on dairy foods.

Grains: bread, cake, biscuits, pizza, pasta
Grains like wheat and oats have a fibrous husk (bran) and a small protein-rich germ. The rest, the endosperm, is pure starch. Starch makes up over 80% of a wheat grain and starch is, of course, a carb made from chains of glucose; a pre-sugar, if you like. Before modern milling, flour was wholemeal and wholegrain and because the germ didn't keep for long, it deteriorated quickly. The modern bleached white stuff is germ free, almost totally carbohydrate and lasts pretty well indefinitely. The list of grain-based foods is exceedingly long, but four of my Big-6 carbs are grains or are grain derived (bread, pizza, pasta, rice). If you have diabetes or pre-diabetes or are overweight, grain/flour-based products are very likely to be part of your problem. So, I am really very

sorry to say this, biscuits, cakes, crispy snacks, pastries, bagels, croutons... all lovely but all starchy, which means they are full of high-energy carbs. Avoid, even if they are promoted as a slow-burn complex-carbohydrate. Your stomach is a very efficient incinerator when it comes to any grain-based food, slow-burn or not but guess what? Life can go on with bread, or even cake. Let them eat vegetables? If you must have it, then eat it; but small portions please, an occasional treat. Again, if you must have them frequently, then stop reading now and give this book to someone else.

Rice
That S-word again. Another starchy grain. Small portions, occasional servings but why, you may ask, are Chinese and other Oriental peoples usually very slim, despite eating so much rice? I am sure there are a number of reasons, not least of which is that they tend to cook real food from raw ingredients to go with it. They also tend to eat far less than the average European too; at least they used to. East Asian cuisine involves real cooking, real food and modest portions. This was the case until recently, but things are, I fear, starting to change. Fast food has gone east. Another reason may have been the historical absence of sugar in oriental diets. Because it liberates fructose during digestion, table sugar in anything more than small amounts can trigger an insulin resistant state after which starchy carbs feed the flames and keep it going. More on fructose later.

Vegetables
All true vegetables are fine. It just depends what you call a true vegetable. Some people simplify it by saying anything that grows above ground is fine whereas roots and tubers that grow underground are not. Roots and tubers are, of course, a cunning plant-like way of storing energy (in the form of our old friend starch) and then hiding it out of sight. So, it won't come as a surprise to learn that potatoes, sweet potato, yams and, to a lesser extent parsnips, are high-carb vegetables. Jerusalem artichokes, carrots and beetroot are medium-carb roots. Everything else, from asparagus to tomatoes and even turnips, surprisingly, are low-carb foods that are fine to cook

with and eat. So, boil, bake, shred, stir-fry, steam or spiralise them; you may even eat some of them raw. Potatoes are the big exception. Avoid combining low-carb veg with other high-carb foods. Again, all pretty obvious.

Potato and the root vegetables

Propaganda posters in the Second World War declared that 'Potato Pete' is an energy food. Citizens in the UK and elsewhere were encouraged to Dig for Victory and dig they did. Up came their lawns and flower beds and planted instead were potatoes. Food energy was in short supply and potatoes are packed with carby energy, and that energy is starch. The potato plant stashes energy away underground for a rainy day, then we come along, dig them up and steal it. A few plants can make fatty compounds, olives and avocados for example, but most are set up to store their energy as starch. For many the root system seems to be the preferred place to put it. 'Boil 'em, mash 'em, stick 'em in a stew', was one cook's advice[4]. Tasty perhaps but dangerous for the diabetic. I like chips, but only have them two or three times a year now – a very occasional treat, part of a feast rather than one of my staples. Come to think of it, I do love roasties, boiled new potatoes, baked spuds and mash too but I just know that my body chemistry is way too sensitive to the starch-sugar-glucose thing for me to eat any of them except once in a blue moon.

Beans, Pulses and Legumes

Légumes (with an accent) is the French word for vegetables. However, the English word legume refers just to bean-pod producing plants, many of which can be used to add nitrogen to the soil. Pulses are the dried fruits of leguminous plants; dried beans, in other words. The number of beans out there is vast and includes chickpeas, peanuts, haricot beans, kidney beans, soya beans, garden peas, French beans, mange tout and lentils. Most are protein rich but also deliver around 15-20% carbs by weight. The carb content varies greatly from bean to bean, so it is useful to check a carb-counter reference and then be modest with portion sizes. The precise carb content of any food ingredient becomes particularly important if you need to count carbs to get your chemistry corrected. Good news; most people manage fine without having to go that far. More about carb counting, if you are interested, later. Note: peanuts are legumes, not true nuts. You can find more information about them in Appendix 2.

Fruit and Berries

Our stone-age antecedents may well have gorged on fruit – but two things: fruit way back then was fibrous stuff. It may have hung low, but it would not have tasted very sweet to our modern pampered palates. Secondly, it came but in season. Ancient fruit, with its meagre motherload of sugar, was a very infrequent treat. Today, after centuries of horticultural improvement, fruit is bigger, juicier and sweeter than ever before in history. That's right; we humans have been doing genetic modification for centuries. Our stone-age forefathers probably wouldn't even recognise the stuff we consider 'natural' now. Also, with international supply lines, that seasonal tie is long gone. The only seasonal variation that remains today is the price.

Most fruits today pack a serious sugary punch and yet fruit is perceived generally as a totally natural and health-promoting food. In fact, it is in my view neither, though I do have to concede that it does taste good. *Beating Diabetes* says fruit is in reality a serious glucose-fructose sugar hitter. The only reason to eat fruit is because it is an enjoyable treat. True, there is some fibre in fruit but there is way more fibre in vegetables. There is vitamin C in fruit but lots, as it happens, in many other foods too. Fruit contains precious few other vitamins or minerals, with the exception in some cases of potassium. So, what to do about fruit? Well, if you desire it, then eat some but maybe just one piece. You may enjoy eating an orange, or even two but you would need to press four or five oranges to get one glassful of juice and that juice will contain all the sugar but very little of the fibre present in the original whole fruit. So ignore the propaganda.

Fruit is a sugar-dense food. Fruit is not a health food. It is sweet and juicy for a reason - sugar. Eat it if you enjoy it but eat it whole. So no smoothies, no fruit juices, no fruit in syrup or sprinkling it with sugar either. Aim for a maximum of one small portion per day. Only eat fruit for pleasure, not health. Oh and a special word about dried fruit. It has all the sugar and none of the water, which for fresh fruit is usually quite a lot. The result is that dried fruit is a much denser sugar source. Grapes, for example, are very high in sugar to start with but, when dried (raisins) are, weight for weight significantly higher in sugar than the fresh fruit. The same goes for dried apricots, prunes and other dried fruits too. In short, in prehistoric times we did the bidding of fruit-bearing plants. We ate their offerings to spread their seeds. Today the tables have turned. Plants now do as we bid and deliver us sweetness and, in many cases, their fruits are sterile so no seed to spread.

Berries are different in one important particular. They contain less sugar weight for weight than regular fruit. So, blueberries, blackberries, strawberries and, in particular, raspberries are good. A small handful, two or three times a week is fine. Again, eat them whole. No juicing. See Appendix 3 for some juicy fruity data.

Nuts, herbs and spices
A carb breakdown of various nuts can be found in Appendix 2. Basically, a small handful of nuts as a snack, or garnish on your food, is good but perhaps be cautious with cashews. They are surprisingly quite high in carbs. Chestnuts are even higher. There is no restriction on using any herbs or spices as long as they are not adulterated with syrups or hidden sugars and starches.

Sugar and fructose
The ultimate nutrition-free edible product. It's hidden in almost every processed food you buy now, even bran flakes and muesli. Read food labels, hunt it down and assiduously avoid. Look out for weasel ways of sneaking sugars into foods without mentioning them directly on the label – dextrose, fructose, corn syrup, agave nectar, honey, to name but five. Sugar is hidden in things like tomato ketchup, non-diet cola

drinks and many cocktails, even sausages and, of course, it is the main ingredient in confectionery.

Sugar and by that I mean sucrose or table sugar, has even been promoted as a weight loss product. The thinking behind this fallacy is that sucrose has a low glycaemic-index (GI). It does not produce as big a surge in blood glucose as, for example, the equivalent amount of bread or potato. Although this is true, it is only half the story, literally, as sucrose is only half glucose. The other half is fructose, which does not get turned into glucose during digestion. Sucrose has a low-GI because it ignores the fructose component (of which more below).

You may encounter products promoted as having 'no added sugars'. This is a sneaky way of saying that the food naturally contained sugar in the first place. A good example again is fruit. It does not mean it is sugar-free or low-carb as almost always it is high-carb. I saw a van selling fruit-slushes and smoothies for children recently. Guess what? It proclaimed they had no added sugar. Of course they didn't. This is technically true but the subliminal selling message being peddled was 'no sugar here' and that was most definitely not the case. So, if the product says it has no *added* sugar, it almost always means there was already plenty in it to start with. Nutritionists and dieticians call this intrinsic sugar as opposed to extrinsic or added sugar.

Sucrose is also the sugar we enjoy when we eat fruit. It is the fructose bit in the fruit that makes it so sweet and tells us it's ripe. The only common exception is bananas, which are made of starch mostly and mainly liberate glucose during digestion. There is very little fructose in bananas. Modern fruit packs a lot of sucrose and therefore a lot of fructose gets released during digestion too.

Sucrose (table sugar) is a double sugar molecule. It's half fructose, half glucose. Fructose, also known as fruit sugar, is much sweeter than glucose. Fructose does occur naturally as a single sugar in small amounts in some fruits, honey and, curiously, seminal fluid. In commercial products like fizzy drinks, fructose is the main sweetener. The fructose manufacturing process usually involves taking starch from corn, breaking it down into glucose, then chemically transforming it to fructose. The fructose-rich liquor is then cut with liquid glucose to make high-fructose corn syrup. This, dear reader, is not something you can do in your own kitchen. The combination used in most regular sodas is HFCS 55, which is 55% fructose, 45% glucose; not very different from the proportions found in regular sucrose but just that little bit sweeter. Glucose is metabolised around the body to provide energy and to replenish glycogen stores. Anything in excess of immediate requirements is transformed into fat and stored. Fructose is different. It is a sugar but, unlike glucose, it has virtually no effect on insulin. It can only really be metabolised in the liver. Unfortunately, the liver has only a very small capacity for dealing with fructose and when that capacity is exceeded, it converts the excess to fat and stores it locally. Over time, fructose consumption can lead to something called a fatty liver and even a fatty pancreas. These conditions contribute significantly to our old friend insulin resistance (Figure 3.3). Fructose in anything other than small amounts is a health hazard. Avoid, avoid. I say again, avoid!

Confectionery
Confectionery is sugar, literally in-your-face sugar. Sugar can be hidden away in so many foods. It can be a natural 'intrinsic' component in many others (which can then be advertised as 'no added sugar' products) but confectionery makes no pretence about what it is. It is sweet oral sugary gratification. It feeds the addiction. In my opinion, it has almost no nutritional qualities. I don't think this can come as much of a surprise to anyone but it is diabetic dynamite. Avoid, avoid, and I say, yet again, avoid.

Energy drinks
I am sorry to do this to you but have a peep at your waistline. I am guessing that most of you will see something just a little more ample than ideal? Yes, we are talking fat. Energy-dense

fat, stored away for that rainy day, the rainy day that never seems to come. So, do you really think you need an energy drink? All a glucose or sucrose energy drink will do is become body-fuel and immediately block any chance of fat burning. You cannot burn fat in the presence of glucose and insulin. Energy drinks, therefore, block fat release/weight loss. In my humble view and we are all allowed a view surely, is that they are a scam and a *diabesity* promoting scam at that. See discussion of energy sources and how to use them in Chapter 6 - Fast.

Alcohol
Wine is fine in moderation, as long as it's dry, not sweet. Champagne, they say, of all the wines, has the lowest effect on blood sugar. Prosecco is similar. Spirits have no direct effect on blood sugar at all, but because of their potency should be enjoyed only occasionally. Beer, stout, porter, lager, cider, perry and other brewed drinks are a whole different kettle of fish. Unlike wine, beers and lagers are made from malted barley and malt (or maltose to give it its proper name) is a sugar. Maltose, like sucrose, is a double sugar but, unlike sucrose, it is made of two glucose molecules joined at the hip. I like a pint myself but it is a very occasional treat now and not a regular thing. There are, of course, many other alcohol-containing drinks. Port and sherry deliver a bigger sugar hit than wine and cocktails are often higher still. Alcopops appeal to younger drinkers, particularly because of their high sugar content and must be avoided. See Appendix 5 for further data on alcohol.

Oils and fats
These are all zero carb and, as such, you might expect me to just say use and enjoy any of them. Sadly, no. In case you missed it earlier, there is a section near the top of this chapter describing the high Omega-6 content of the industrially extracted seed oils (rapeseed, sunflower, soya safflower etc.). Natural vegetable oils like olive and avocado oil are obtained by crushing or centrifuging the fruit. Getting oil out of rape, canola or soya beans seeds, for example, is usually a heavy industrial operation involving a sequence of chemical

processes. Natural this ain't. So stick with the natural ones and avoid the high Omega-6 vegetable oils. Note: Even when cold pressed, seed/vegetable oils are high in Omega-6 fats, (see Appendix 1 for more detailed information) stick to and indeed enjoy regularly and liberally, natural fats and oils like butter, lard, suet and olive oil.

Sweeteners

I feel a bit conflicted about the non-caloric sweeteners and have done so for quite some time. They are sweet, they are zero-calorie, so surely that must be good, right? Hmmm. I really am unsure about this. Firstly, with perhaps the exception of stevia, they are not real foods. They are by-products of the chemical industry. It seems their sweet qualities were mostly found by accident. The internet is more than usually awash with virulent argument both for and against. I do, however, buy the idea that using sweeteners just keeps one's sweet cravings going. It excuses users from letting their palates adapt to the taste and qualities of real food. There are even plausible arguments that the sweet taste has brain-chemistry effects similar to those evoked by regular sugar. Brain chemistry is what addiction is all about. Artificial sweeteners may even disturb the balance of bugs in our bowel, our microbiome. The biggest concern I have is that they may stimulate insulin secretion. Why? Well when we taste their (artificial) sweetness in our mouths, the body may secrete insulin in preparation for an expected glucose surge that never comes. The hip phrase for this is the *cephalic insulin response*, or what your brain starts doing when it suspects a sugar hit is on the way. Stevia may be a little different. It is harvested from nature. Its leaves have been used for hundreds of years as a sweetener in beverages in South America but for me, about all other sweeteners, the jury is out for the time being. However, any industrially produced edible substance just has to be suspect, even if it's zero-cal. I suspect it will not be long before the jury returns to deliver their verdict and I am expecting it to be 'guilty, m' lud'.

A few words about... pick a number between 5 and 10 a day

Having read my rather negative piece on high-fructose tree-candy (aka fruit), the question that might pop into your mind is 'If fruit has precious little minerals and virtually no vitamins other than vitamin C and if it can tip significant amounts of sugar into our bloodstream, why do our Official guidelines push it so hard?' Sadly, I am afraid that the answer is, I suspect, that our Official dietary advisers have been conditioned, nay groomed, into believing that fruit is the cornerstone of a healthy diet. Well, guess what, there are no essential carbohydrates, not one. Even if they look and taste good, even if they are juicy, fresh and sweet, they are, in fact, (from a nutritional and dietary point of view) just treats or fun foods. Bearing in mind the wallop of sugar most of them deliver, they really are something to be cautious about. I am not knocking their place as enjoyable items to eat but consider this, until the development of modern transport and preservation technology, fruit was only ever a brief seasonal treat. There were apples in the autumn, satsumas at Christmas. Fruit has only very recently become a commodity with all-year-round availability.

You may think using the words 'conditioning' and 'grooming' are a little harsh. I'm sure our Official diet experts would but I don't. It seems that most them are as much victims of one of the most successful marketing strategies of recent times – the 5-a-day campaign but have you ever wondered where the 5-a-day slogan came from?

The surprising truth is that the '5-a-day for better health' idea was conceived in 1988 as a social marketing enterprise by the Californian Department of Health Services[5]. The slogan only really took off in 1991 when it was endorsed by an organisation called the Produce for Better Health Foundation. This organisation was funded by a large number of organisations that grow or market fresh produce, from The Agroamerica Fruit Company to Zespri Kiwifruit. Its role is to advocate for the fruit and vegetable growers of America[6]. Now why would fruit growers endorse the 5-a-day thing? You may well ask. Since then it has grown like crazy. Every US state now has a 5-a-day coordinator. The slogan was taken up in a big way in the UK in 2003 and has morphed quickly into *at 'least* 5-a-day'. If five is good, is six better? The BBC recently weighed in, reporting on the then latest study '7-a-day fruit and veg 'saves lives''[7]. That ain't the truth either. Fruit in the diet has not been shown conclusively to reduce heart attacks and it has not been shown in large studies to reduce cancer either. So basically, bottom line is, it looks good, it tastes good and, by God… that's about it.

One large study looking at links between fruit consumption and cancer was conducted among almost half a million people in Europe. Over an eight year period, the crude figures showed a small, weak association between fruit intake and lower levels of cancer but the study authors couldn't distinguish between a true effect and the effects of bias (always an issue with observational studies). Walter Willett, one of the world's leading nutritional epidemiologists and renowned low-carb sceptic, commenting on the paper could only say that the weak association was possibly the result of confounding. In summary, he wrote '*the findings from the [study] add further evidence that a broad effort to increase consumption of fruits and vegetables will not have a major effect on cancer incidence.*' Translating that jargon into plain-speak, all this means is that we cannot say, even in a large study with vast numbers of subjects, observed over a very long period, that fruit eating had any effect on cancer rates.

The massive Nurses' Health Study run by Willett's Harvard Department of Nutrition[5] looked at, amongst many other things, the relationship between fruit consumption and the risk of developing Type-2 Diabetes. Their findings showed very weak beneficial associations with suggestions that berries may be more protective. Again, as ever in these large nutritional studies, an observational approach was necessary, so the small associations between fruit eating and a lower incidence of diabetes proved nothing. Association can never prove causation. They concluded *Total fruit consumption is not consistently associated with a lower risk of Type-2 Diabetes*[9]. Plus, one of the authors admitted *Residual or unmeasured or residual confounding may still exist.* This certainly wasn't a ringing endorsement for eating fruit as a health option either. In the discussion section of the paper, the authors did acknowledge the great variability in research findings among the various other studies done on this subject. Basically, the question is whether fruit eaters tend to be naturally healthier people and less cancer prone than those who choose not to eat fruit? My hunch is, yes, they may very well be.

The truth is, we have been conditioned to believe 5-a-day is healthy and 'we' includes many of our Official dietary guideline writers. For them it is a no-brainer, so obvious that it is not worth thinking about. Fruit, they believe, is better than pills and much tastier too but the closer you look, the more apparent it becomes that it is vegetables and not fruit, that should be the bulk of any five portions. From an evolutionary perspective, fruit is a prize. Its only job is to lure us into doing something for a tree. Combine that with several thousand years of horticultural improvement and what we now get from the fresh fruit aisle at the supermarket, it really is sugary tree-candy. So, choose vegetables rather than fruit. They provide minerals, vitamins and fibre too and, unlike fruit, most vegetables are not stuffed with glucose and they do not deliver a whack of fructose either. One portion of fruit a day, should you wish to enjoy it, is quite enough for anyone. Oh and as for classing fruit pies and jam as part of your 5-a-day; no comment necessary... I hope.

A word about carb cutting
The cutting of carbs is a subject we will return to properly in 'Fail', a chapter towards the end of the book but at this stage a couple of pointers might be useful.

First: the intensity of the carb-cutting required to correct the body's chemistry and move it away from its diabetic insulin-domination, will vary from person to person. For some, simply removing added 'extrinsic' or added sugars from the diet might suffice but for most of us with diabetes, Step Three on the ladder below (Table 3.4) will be required to reverse insulin's domination of the body. For those who are more intensely carbohydrate intolerant, a virtually zero-carb approach may be necessary, at least for a while. Table 3.4 describes the various levels or intensities of carb-restriction that may be required. Do not at this stage get too hung up on details, just let the concept seep into your consciousness.

Second: In Chapter 4 - Cook, you will find some specimen menus presenting the sorts of meals that can work well if you are trying to beat your diabetes. For the time being, *Beating Diabetes* majors on choosing ingredients wisely and, as we shall see, aiming to rustle up lovely menus. The whole science of targets for how many grams of carb you should aim for is only relevant if the ingredient/meal choices approach of *Shop, Cook, Dine* does not produce the desired result for you.

One of the things people with Type-1 Diabetes can do to make life easier for themselves is to attend a DAFNE course. On it they will be given very useful and practical advice about how to manage their food and insulin requirements more efficiently. In effect, it enables them to push their insulin doses up and down, depending on what they choose to eat, in the same way a non-diabetic person is able to do naturally. DAFNE stands for Dose Adjustment For Normal Eating. I suppose *Beating Diabetes* turns this concept around and suggests Food Adjustment for the Normal New You. Now there is a potential acronym that will never catch on but the point is, for people with Type-2 Diabetes or pre-diabetes, changing what you eat may be a more logical response to a carb-insulin-driven disorder than the alternative; taking medication to try and control the carb-driven problem.

Conclusion
Let us check where we are. In Chapter 2, the 'How to get Type-2 Diabetes?' chapter, you discovered... how you got diabetes. Diabetes is a condition caused and propelled by eating sugary and starchy carbs. Some people can cope with a high-carb diet and even flourish on it, but many cannot. The medical and nutritional establishments, however, see diabetes as the consequence of overeating and under exercising. Too many calories in, too few out; gluttony and sloth, to use

pejorative and unkind words. Obesity, in their view, is the cause of diabetes. In fact, we have discovered something different, that obesity and diabetes are the direct result of the disturbed carb-insulin combo. It's not the calories, it's a chemistry thing. Dr Robert Lustig is a paediatric endocrinologist and medical writer. He sees and treats children with a range of hormonal conditions, one of which is obesity (yes, obesity is a hormonal condition). Increasingly of late, he has been seeing more cases of Type-2 Diabetes in adolescents. He is a prolific writer and perhaps the United States' leading campaigner against sugar. He would prefer to see diabetes renamed. His suggestion is 'Processed Food Disease'[10].

Which brings us nicely back to where we started this chapter. In it, most of the common foods were neatly divided into two groups; the ones you can eat, drink, be merry and remain healthy on (the In-Foods list) and the others that those who have diabetes should avoid, eschew and reject for the restoration of their health (the Out-Foods list). The lists mainly, though not exclusively, describe real food ingredients, not processed foods, not chemicals. Time now to move on and think about what we can do with those lovely In-Foods ingredients. Let the cooking begin.

Table 3.4: How to cut your carbs – a ladder of possibilities

Step 1	Cut out added "extrinsic" sugars	The easy first step in reducing you sugar-insulin combo's domination. Cut down/out sugar in tea or coffee, sugar incorporated into your cooking, or sprinkled on strawberries, and of course in confectionery. The number of potential sugar-hits lurking out there is vast.
Step 2	Cut out hidden "intrinsic" sugars	Step 1 plus... cut down/out naturally sugary foods, the ones which may be advertised as 'no added sugar'. So, fruit in all its forms, from whole fruit, to dried fruit, smoothies and puree, would be prime examples.
Step 3	Cut out potent starchy carbs as well	Steps 1 and 2 plus...cut down/out on grains and floury foods like bread, pasta, cake, biscuits, rice. Also cut down/out starchy foods like potato. This includes hidden starches, for example those in many sauces and in most processed foods. Fear not - there is plenty left you can eat with pleasure.
Step 4	Cut out all starchy carbs	Steps 1-3 plus... cut out all of the above, but also moderate-carb carb foods like pulses and legumes and dairy products with milk-sugar in them. The sugar surge after so-called zero-carb meals should be miniscule.

Notes:

(1) A quotation attributed to Hippocrates, the Father of Medicine.
https://www.goodreads.com/author/quotes/248774.Hippocrates

(2) A fantastic site packed with high quality advice and resources. **https://www.dietdoctor.com**

(3) The Pioppi Diet. Aseem Malhotra and Donal O'Neill. Penguin Books

(4) A quotation attributed to the hobbit Sam Gamgee. It features in Peter Jackson's film but not in the original book written by JRR Tolkien.
https://www.youtube.com/watch?v=a8ZelsfYAb0&list=RDa8ZelsfYAb0&start_radio=1&t=53.

(5) **https://www.sciencedirect.com/science/article/pii/S0749379718304884**

(6) For an excellent article on the subject go to this link on Dr Zoë Harcombe's web page.

http://www.zoeharcombe.com/2012/03/five-a-day-the-truth/

(7) https://www.bbc.co.uk/news/health-26818377

(8) Department of Nutrition at the Harvard T.H. Chan School of Public Health **https://www.hsph.harvard.edu/nutrition/**

(9) https://www.bmj.com/content/347/bmj.f5001

(10) http://www.robertlustig.com/processed-food/

Chapter 4 – Cook

A real meal revolution

So where have we got to? Well, we have identified the Number one metabolic disturbance underlying and driving diabetes – excessive secretion of the hormone insulin aided and abetted by its partner in crime, insulin resistance. We know that for many of us, diabetes is the consequence of a high-carb diet. We also know that correcting that body-chemistry defect is quite simple, at least in theory: cut the high-energy carbs – the Big-6 of bread, pasta, pizza, rice, potato and sugar. Cut them and immediately, on Day-1, you will cut blood glucose surges. Cut the surges and you will cut insulin secretion and, as you will no doubt recall from Chapter 1 *Welcome to Planet Diabetes*, it is difficult to store fat in the absence of insulin and you cannot release fat in its presence. Insulin makes you fat, insulin keeps you fat, oh... and a disturbed insulin balance is also the main driver for Type-2 Diabetes.

In the last chapter, foods were neatly divided into two groups; those that have virtually no effect on your blood sugar or insulin levels and those that push levels up high; the In-Foods and Out-Foods, in other words. To be true to the ethos of *Beating Diabetes* (focusing on food, not chemistry), we should now at last look, not at Official nutritional advice, nor at published Recommended Daily Allowances, nor even at the dark arts of food labels and traffic-light advisories. No, we should now think about real menus. So, let us look at a variety of real meals, the sort that low-carb dining is all about. I know that they are real meals because they are ones I cook regularly myself.

Below you will find sections on
- Breakfast suggestions
- Salad dishes
- Soups (homemade, of course)

- Meat dishes
- Offal dishes
- Fish dishes
- Vegetarian dishes and…
- Desserts

There are, of course, hundreds, even thousands, of low-carb meals out there. The internet is replete with them. If you have not been a low-carber previously, you are going to have to start somewhere. So why not start with me in my kitchen, with what I tend to eat regularly and enjoy?

This section is more about menus than recipes. Brief recipes are suggested but bookshops both real and virtual, any number of TV programmes and, of course, the internet, are stuffed with advice on how to prepare all these kinds of meals. There are usually several different ways to prepare any one meal. Just find one that works for you, taking care to avoid studiously the potent carbohydrate foods; the starchy and sugary ones, in other words.

I have listed a number of general menu suggestions but only one designated meal in particular; that tricky little first meal of the day called breakfast. Other menu suggestions are grouped under meal types. So, there are soups, there are salads, there are meat, fish and vegetarian dishes and there are even some dessert suggestions too, yes there really are some low-carb desserts out there.

For most meal types, I have aimed to present seven suggestions, simply because there are seven days in the week. After all, you do not want to get bored. Although these are all meals I regularly prepare and enjoy myself, it will be obvious I am neither a chef nor a committed foodie. The meals described here are suggestions for regular daily fare, not dinner parties. The meals are all easy to prepare and do not require exotic ingredients, sophisticated kitchen equipment, or great culinary skill. They are all *Beating Diabetes* compliant;

they are low-carb offerings, in other words. This is *Beating Diabetes* in your kitchen, in real life.

We are, of course, all sinners in this fallen world. We all fall short but there is good news. These suggestions are meant to present staple meals, ones on which you can subsist regularly. The occasional sinful feast or naughty indulgence is not the end of the world. Make sure you enjoy them thoroughly when you stray but do make sure to return to the stable of staples afterwards.

Breakfast

•   **Omelettes:** I am a great fan of eggs. Boiled, poached, scrambled or fried. Omelettes should be cooked quickly and are great filled, folded and flipped. My filling choices include things like cooked mushrooms, shredded spring onions, strips of ham or salmon and, of course, cheese. You can toss some herbs in too; basil or chives, for example, are lovely. Serve on a warmed plate (if you have time) and season with pepper and a dash of salt. Perhaps have some of the fillings prepped the night before sitting in the fridge.

•   **Egg on wilted spinach:** Scrambled eggs are different. Whip them up with a fork and a dash of milk and cook slowly, turning the eggy mix over and over. You could throw in some chives or salmon bits, even thin slices of ham. Dot with a knob of butter then transfer the hot scrambled eggs on to a warm plate. Season and enjoy. Actually, I prefer poached eggs on my spinach these days. Throw your spinach leaves into a little boiling water, stir and cover and, within two minutes they are done. Meanwhile, crack the egg into a small bowl and slip it into hot but not boiling water (bubbling messes up the shape). Try and serve with the golden yoke still soft. Then grind that pepper. Adding a spoonful of chunky homemade tomato sauce makes this a more substantial meal. Strain or sieve the spinach to get any watery juice out, transfer immediately on to a warmed plate, then lay your eggs on top. This meal is one you can do some prep work for in advance. Wilted drained spinach and tomato sauce can be prepared the day before and microwaved as your egg cooks.

•   **The Full English:** Not something I sit down to every day, or even every week, but a substantial cooked breakfast is a delight. I usually cook it for others rather than myself. I like to do the cooking and serving so that my guests can concentrate on dining without distraction. So, crispy bacon, black pudding (check the food label for starchy fillers like oats, maybe even a sausage or two (again check that info box for lurking carbs), fried mushroom (in butter) and cooked tomato. All washed down with a mug of tea (no sugar). Fab, but... no toast, no fried bread, no hash browns, no potato wedges. Keep it low-carb and you will not slide into insulin domination and you will continue to feel full, immune to temptation, way past elevenses. Vegetarians can of course omit the offending meaty ingredients and perhaps sub in something of their own from the In-Foods list. Warning: the full English is a bit of a calorie bomb and perhaps not a good choice when you first go low-carb. In that first week or three, modesty with portion sizes is helpful.

•   **A Suffolk Breakfast Smörgåsbord:** You probably guessed I made this up but sometimes a selection of cheeses, gravadlax (surprisingly easy to make yourself at home) or smoked salmon, meats (ham, pastrami, chicken) and salamis, served with crudités (sticks of raw carrot, bell pepper, cucumber, celery, broccoli or cauliflower) with perhaps olives and hummus makes a nice low-carb change. Not cheap and not a quick dash-for-the-door breakfast, this one. An occasional treat; more one to share and dine over on a day off.

•   **Mushrooms and sausages**: Make sure you check what is in your sausages. Some of the more flavoured ones come with a sneaky hidden slug of sugars and others might be bulked out with fillers like starchy rusk. Mushrooms always seem to be tastier if fried in butter. Whenever I have tried to fry them in vegetable oil, they seem to act like blotting paper and, of course, vegetable oils are Omega-6 heavy and to be avoided (See Appendix 1). How about tomatoes on the side, or even baked beans? I wish I hadn't mentioned baked beans there. They are a bit of a conundrum. Homemade ones may be fine, but the process is more than a little tedious.

Fruit and yoghurt: If you like fruit, then eat some. Actually, in my view, there is no other reason to eat fruit. If you do choose to indulge in fruit, go for a whole piece of fruit and not a fruit drink (sugar in a fruity disguise) or a smoothie (lots of sugar in a fruity disguise). I have a hunch that preceding or following a carby-meal, like ones containing fruit, with physical exercise may slightly reduce the food's adverse effect on blood glucose and insulin levels. Why? Well muscular activity burns glucose, much of which comes from its in-house energy store, glycogen. Some of the blood glucose surge, after eating an apple, say, will then be diverted into your muscle cells to replenish their glycogen stores. Unfortunately, most fruit also gives your system a whack of fructose as well as glucose (starchy bananas are an exception; they liberate mostly glucose alone). Yoghurt, of course, can be a sugary Trojan horse. Read the label and remember if it brags about being 'low-fat' it is very probably high-sugar. Or if it boasts 'no added sugar' it is likely to be '*intrinsic*' sugary-fruit heavy. Anyway, a tub of yoghurt and a piece of fruit, or even better a small handful of berries like raspberries or blueberries, are nice once in a while. A small word of warning though, a low-fat, low-protein breakfast like fruit with yoghurt isn't going to keep you full for long. See Appendix 3 for some fruity facts that may help you decide which to choose for your indulgence.

Yesterday's leftovers: I am making a big assumption here; and it is that yesterday's food was *Beating Diabetes* compliant. If it was, then it will be fine for breakfast too. Of course, some of us may find reheating a bowl of chicken casserole, or some leftover lamb Madras a tad disturbing at seven-thirty in the morning but that is only because we have been groomed over a lifetime to believe that breakfast equals carbs and that cereals and fruit are somehow the only right and proper options for our morning fodder. Let's face it, most modern breakfasts have more in common with puddings and desserts these days. So, emancipate yourself from breakfast slavery. Throw off your high-carb chains, I say and eat free.

• **Niçoise salad**: I like this one partially because of the mix of textures and flavours but also because, with a little forethought, it can be assembled and ready to eat in five minutes. My current ingredient list is tinned tuna (in water, brine or olive oil, not sunflower oil), Kalamata olives, capers, shredded spring onion, cherry tomato halves and egg quarters, all on a bed of shredded lettuce and dressed with a lemony vinaigrette. Mmmm, low-carb, almost sugar-free and lovely. A crumbling of feta is nice but may come with a small carb-consequence.

• **Egg (or even tuna) mayo:** two other quickies. Check the mayo is not a sneaky carb or vegetable oil loaded imposter. There are helpful videos on the net showing how to make real Omega-6-free mayo. Garnish the eggy mix with a dusting of cayenne and some chopped spring onion, then serve on a bed of leaves. My tuna mayo usually sports a bit of fresh grated ginger too.

• **Pea, bean and garlic salad:** This is one Bev usually does for me. Briefly blitz up the cooked garden peas with a hint or two of garlic. Stir into cooked broad beans. Serve cold with a topping of grated Parmesan on a bed of leaves with a vinaigrette of your choice. This is a slightly naughty dish. Peas and beans are pulses and are around 10% and 16% carb, respectively. Brisk walks before and/or after will help clear the glucose surge.

• **Asparagus in Parma ham salad:** Asparagus farms surround my house and the local stuff is great boiled, steamed, baked or even fried. I like wrapping the spears tightly in Parma ham, dousing them with some olive oil, then baking till the Parma crisps up. Serve hot with a green salad. A few shaves of parmesan cheese on top sets the plate off nicely.

• **Coleslaw salad:** There are so many variations on this theme. I like chopped white onion, a mix of red and savoy cabbage with carrot, all raw. I might add grain mustard and mayonnaise and a little sour cream, or even a spoonful of horseradish sauce. I think a bit of a vinegary hit helps too. Dollop it on to anything you like, or have it with some lamb's lettuce.

• **A ploughman's with pickles**: Not a salad I do very often but one I enjoy when I get around to it. Sliced ham, boiled egg, cheddar cheese, a few tomatoes and a sprig or two of something green. A spoonful of coleslaw is nice with it too and, if you like, a gherkin or a pickled onion but... no scotch egg, no pork pie. Keep the Big-6 carbs out.

• **A basic green salad:** Not so much a salad meal but rather an almost universal accompanying side order. Lettuce of course, matchsticks of spring onion, perhaps a few thin strips of green pepper, or celery. Dress with a blob of mayo or a dash of vinaigrette and you are done. You can boost it with nuts or avocado. Sometimes a few slivers of crunchy apply are nice too; not too many, mind. Remember, even apples are tree-candy. The basic green salad goes particularly nicely with fish or a ploughman's. A great way to present the salad is dusted with a generous layer of freshly grated parmesan cheese.

Soups

• **Tomato soup.** Fry onions, carrots and celery in butter. Toss in skinned tomatoes followed by tinned plum tomatoes and either some passata or tomato puree. Simmer for a few minutes then break it all up with a hand blender or in a food processor. Serve with a dash or Worcestershire sauce (or even better Henderson's Relish) and a sprig of basil. These tomato products contain a small amount of carbohydrate. Check the food labels for its carb content and perhaps factor in a little strategic exercise to create a glycogen deficit. That way any glucose will be mopped up by muscles rather than vanishing straight into your fat stores (see the Exercise chapter).

• **Onion Soup.** Shred onions, fry in butter and add hot stock. When cooked, garnish with grated cheese (Gruyère is traditional) but omit the floating slice of bread.

• **Carrot and coriander soup.** Fry some shredded onions and add in your diced carrots. Frazzle for 3-4 minutes then throw in most of the coriander (chopped up) followed by vegetable stock. Boil then blend to the consistency you wish. Season and serve with a few fronds of coriander on top.

• **Chicken soup.** Make chicken stock. Add chopped vegetables of choice, herbs and shredded chicken meat. Thigh meat is tastier.

• **Pea and mint.** Vegetable stock, peas and mint. Blend to desired consistency. A nice soup to serve cold. Watch out, peas are a bit carby.

- **Mushroom.** Just like tomato soup but throw in chopped-up mushrooms instead. Serve with a splash of cream and a few thin fried mushroom slices on top. Nice.
- **Fish chowder.** I am not a shellfish, crustacean or mollusc-eating sort of person. They don't agree with me, so I omit them (as well as potato, which is a common chowder ingredient). However, I do like the sort of seafood that comes with a face and a few fins. Make a vegetable stock, add herbs (dill or tarragon are nice), perhaps some vegetables, then add cream. Finally add in your bits of bone-free fish (cod, smoked haddock, salmon, monkfish, even). Keep the pot hot for a few minutes while the fish cooks through. Serve into warm bowls with a blob of cream or yoghurt on top and a sprig or two of something green. There does appear to be a bit of a green sprig theme running through this chapter.

Meat dishes

'All flesh is grass' as Isaiah, my favourite Old Testament prophet, once wrote. At least it should be. So, if you like beef, it is best to go for grass-fed variety, despite the premium price. Why? Because corn and soya fed beasts have meat that tends to have a less healthful Omega-6 dominated fat component. Grass-fed cows mimic the traditional more heavily Omega-3 dominated wild meats. See Appendix 1 for more information about fats and oils. Actually, the same applies to farmed salmon too. Not only is wild salmon more Omega-3 rich but the flesh tends to be firmer and tastier and, no surprise, more expensive too. If you feed fish and cattle on stuff they have not evolved to eat, then do not be surprised that their flesh is less healthy.

- **Spanish style pork stew.** Fry some lardons of bacon with chorizo in olive oil, throw some sliced onions (and garlic) into the sizzling red mixture then the chunks of pork. When the meat is browned, transfer everything into a pan and add tomatoes, stoned olives, herbs and mushrooms. Cook it on the hob, or in a slow cooker, or bake in the oven. Some red wine in the mix helps. It always seems to taste even better the next day. Serve with hot In-Food vegetables.

- **Chicken breast in bacon with pesto**. Another quick and easy favourite. Place the breast on some slices of Parma ham (streaky bacon is cheaper and very nice too). Dollop the pesto on the chicken. Wrap the ham or bacon over the top, anoint with oil and bake.
- **Roast leg of lamb.** Great with rosemary and garlic. A good source of leftovers too.
- **Slow cooked lamb 'tagine'.** For me a tagine dish is more about the North African flavours than the cone-shaped cooking vessel. Cook the lamb slowly with plenty of tomatoes and some harissa paste. A few dried apricots are nice for authenticity but they do add significantly to the carb-load. Garnish with flaked almonds and fresh herbs. Great with a green salad and the leftovers are even tastier next day. Harissa, like tomato, contains a small amount of carbohydrate.
- **Roast chicken.** An absolute standard. Makes an easy main meal with enough leftovers for a chicken salad for tomorrow's lunch. Of course the bones and other bits can be used to make chicken stock. A triple whammy meal deal.
- **Homemade burgers** (or meatballs). If you make your burgers yourself then you will know exactly what is in them. Many recipes include cereals like oats or crunched-up crackers in the mix or even potato starch. I don't follow these. I just use minced beef, minced onions, herbs and seasoning and bind the squishy mixture with a beaten egg. Ground almond can be used as a binder if you wish. Serve with a choice of the usual BBQ-style toppings; pickles, cheese, bacon, mustard. These do not need a bread bun or a mound of chips on the side to be enjoyed. I do much the same for meatballs except of course they are smaller and not flattened. They are great with a homemade tomato sauce and courgetti.
- **Beef stir-fry.** *Oil-in wok-on*, as one of my favourite Chinese cooks used to suggest[2]. I currently use a small amount of avocado oil, for its high smoke point and perhaps add in some sesame seed oil at the end. Actually, avocado oil is a great stir-fry oil; very low Omega-6, high smoke point. More or less any meat chopped up, doused with Chinese five spice and sizzled will do for a quick stir-fry. Throw in some slices of onion, carrot or pepper, or perhaps some ginger or

garlic. Add a few garden peas and, just before serving, a little sherry then some beansprouts. Splash on a little soy sauce when plated up but, nice though they are, no noodles for me, please.

Offal dishes

• **Liver and walnut.** Fry strips of liver with some lardons or slices of chorizo. Add walnut pieces just before serving. Add some cream and herbs as well if you like. Serve with steamed vegetables, or spoon the combo on to a green salad. A blob of mayo goes well with this.

• **Kidney.** Lamb kidney is lovely. Clean and slice then fry in butter. Do not cook for long or they will turn into small ingots of vulcanised rubber. Season and serve on a hot plate with vegetables and a cream and grain mustard dressing. Quick, cheap, delicious.

• **Slow cooked heart stew:** Dice up trimmed heart; lamb's is nice. Transfer to a slow cooker or large pot for the oven. Fry onions in butter, add other veg as desired; carrots, leeks, peas, perhaps. Throw them into the pot. Don't forget some herbs. Glug in some red wine and water (you could use stock). Cook slowly for several hours. An inexpensive, nutritious, hearty, warming dish.

Fish dishes

• **Griddled salmon with pesto sauce.** Another tasty quickie. One to cook outside, if possible, as griddling indoors can leave a lingering fishy aroma (I use a small cheap gas-powered camping burner). Start skin side up and after you flip the slice of fish over, spoon on the pesto. You could use sun-dried tomatoes instead if you prefer, or both.

• **Salmon and avocado.** Steam the salmon. You could do this with foil parcels or in the microwave. Flake coarsely when cooked and combine with chopped avocado. A spring onion garnish is good. Season, add mayo and incorporate everything gently to preserve the lovely textures. Spoon the mixture gently into the empty avocado skins and serve. A dill or basil garnish is nice.

• **Seared tuna steaks.** Yet another quickie and great

with a lime and coriander dressing (olive oil, lime juice with zest, wine vinegar, chopped coriander. Delia Smith adds garlic, capers and grain mustard to her recipe, which is delicious).

- **Cod in pancetta.** A bit like chicken in Parma ham but this time with fish. Goes very nicely with sun-dried tomatoes too.
- **Sardine stuffed pepper.** Slice the peppers vertically with the stalk carefully cut down its length at one end, then scoop out the seeds and stuff. Fill the pepper 'bowls' with chunks of sardine, fried onions and tomato. Bake. I like capers and a garnish of spring onion and oily sun-dried tomato. Adding in some anchovy makes it even fishier.
- **Bream (or bass) steamed.** Parcel the fillets loosely in aluminium foil. You can add slices of lemon or herbs at this point. Crimp the edges to seal them then bake in the oven. The parcels allow the fish to steam in its own juice. They don't take long to cook.
- **Baked prawns with feta and herbs.** Fry some onions and garlic then add some tinned tomatoes. Heat for a few minutes to reduce and thicken the mixture. Throw in herbs of choice and pour the mixture into an open topped oven-proof dish. Add a layer of prawns and crumbled feta on top and bake for a few minutes until the prawns are cooked through. Garnish with some fresh herbs and serve.

Vegetarian dishes

- **Halloumi cheese with citrus dressing.** Most chefs dust the halloumi slices with flour but I don't bother with that. Fry them in olive oil till a golden crust starts to appear, then flip them over. The same lime and coriander dressing described above for seared tuna is great with this.
- **Stuffed peppers.** Much the same as the sardine recipe above with without the fish. I like garlic and spring onions with the tomatoes and plenty of olive oil.
- **Egg and avocado salad.** Much the same as salmon and avocado but with boiled egg quarters instead. Chives go very well with this meal. A dusting of livid red cayenne on top adds something.

- **Cheesy Ploughman's.** It has to be cheddar, or a similar mature hard cheese. Add a green salad, some celery sticks and a flavoursome tomato or two. You could even throw in a boiled egg as well if you are feeling especially peckish. Add pickles, mustard and mayo and bingo. No bread rolls though.
- **Courgetti with sauce.** I wasn't a fan of courgetti (spiralised courgettes/zucchini) until I discovered that boiling it was the problem. It is so much better when briefly fried in oil (and lardons). Fry it quickly like a stir-fry. The steamed version can easily overcook and turn to mush. For the sauce, make that homemade tomato sauce, (or add minced meat in the cooking to make a ragù. Sorry, veggies). I love puttanesca sauce with courgetti (tomato, chili, basil, anchovy, black olive, garlic and oil, with Parmesan grated on top). If you don't have a spiraliser, you can slice the courgettes with a knife. It just takes longer and the strips come out straight. Note: I find courgetti seems to cook better if after slicing or spiralising it is left to dry out for a few hours (or even overnight).
- **Stuffed aubergine rolls.** Fry or griddle long thinly sliced pieces of aubergine to cook and soften them. When cool, load the thick end of the aubergine slices with feta cheese, some basil leaves and a blob of chunky tomato sauce, then roll 'em up. You may need a cocktail stick to stop the aubergine unrolling. Place them in a tin, season, drizzle with olive oil and bake. The stuffings can be as varied as you wish.
- **Chili 'sans' carne.** Fried onion, carrot, celery, garlic and sweet peppers. Follow with chilli powder then vegetable stock. Add kidney beans and, at the end, the herbs of your choice; basil or coriander perhaps? Blob some cream on top in the bowl. Up to you. Serve with a green salad or cauliflower rice (Google it). Note: Kidney beans are around 23% carb by cooked weight.

Desserts

- **Chocolate mousse.** Separate the yokes from two eggs. Whip egg whites into soft peaks. Melt chocolate (80%) with double cream; careful, don't overheat it. When cooled a

---

little, mix in egg yolks, then fold in the whipped egg white mixture. Pour into small bowls. Cool and serve later. Why not do enough for a few evenings? Garnish with a few berries and some single cream, perhaps.

• **Berries with cream.** Couldn't be simpler. Put some berries in a bowl, raspberries, blackberries, pretty little blueberries, then pour on some cream. Or if you fancy an exciting change, put some thick cream or yoghurt in a bowl and sprinkle the berries on top. Voila! Quick, simple, lovely.

• **Coconut and vanilla ice cream.** You can make this in an ice cream maker if you wish. If not, combine tinned coconut milk (do not use a low-fat variety) with some vanilla extract, non-caloric sweetener of your choice and a pinch of salt. Mix. Transfer to a shallow dish and allow to just freeze a little. Leave it too long and you will have a milky brick on your hands. Remove from freezer, allow it to warm slightly, then break it up. Then, whiz in a food processor and transfer the mixture to a serving dish, before putting it back into the freezer. Best eaten on the day it is made, although it will keep for a week or two.

• **Blueberry sorbet.** Blitz up fresh or frozen berries. Add a little water and a sweetener. Freeze to the point where ice begins to form, then re blitz after breaking up any ice. It has a lovely colour. Some whole fresh blueberries on top looks great.

• **Stewed gooseberries (or rhubarb).** Use a sweetener to counter the tartness, if you like. Serve with cream or ice cream. Hot or cold? It's your call. Bev loves them, but not me. Pass the cheese.

• **Low-carb brownies.** Ground almonds, cacao powder, eggs, butter, chocolate (80%) and some sweetener. Lovely with some berries and single cream. Remarkably filling.

• **Low-carb Eton mess?** This is both possible and tasty, as long as you use sugar-free meringues. You will have to make these yourself. When cooled and dry, break up and mix with some cream and fresh berries.

Conclusion

Okay low-carbers, you now have a few genuine real food meal suggestions. They are specimen meals, examples if you like, not just to be copied but also to inspire you to move deeper into your own low-carb zone and develop your own signature repertoire. Why not use these examples as inspiration for you and your loved ones to adapt your own particular favourites, to make them *Beating Diabetes* and low-carb compliant? In Chapter 3 – Shop, we covered what ingredients to cook with. Here in Cook we have identified a range of easy-to-prepare satisfying meals to enjoy. Next comes Dine. If you are wondering how much better this can get, then read on.

Notes:

(1) For an excellent article on Lenna Cooper and her views on breakfast visit:
https://www.dailytelegraph.com.au/news/how-the-kellogg-brothers-influenced-the-way-westerners-eat-breakfast/news-story/7478e97f93d98c466454ac970a88e9ad

(2) The catch phrase didn't make it into her book *Chinese Food Made easy*. Ching-He Huang. Published by Harper Collins. The spiced beef stir-fry is particularly delicious.

Chapter 5 – Dine

The Ps and Qs of diabetes-friendly dining

'Remove packaging, prick film and microwave on full power for 5 minutes.' This is not cooking; this is just heating something up. Cooking is the skill of preparing a meal from basic ingredients. Cooking means that your food will be 'real' and not industrial, a facsimile that may look and even taste like the real thing but has an ingredient list more like a diabolical chemistry lesson. You know what is in your food if you cook using raw produce rather than buying convenience meals. It can be cheaper too but not always.

Cooking does, of course, take time. There is no getting away from that. Convenience foods, on the other hand, are convenient because they are quick and undemanding. No skill is required other than carefully avoiding a third-degree mouth burn when serving it straight from the microwave. Processed foods and prepared meals are very likely to major on a large number of chemical additives but a very small range of food ingredients. These food products are usually potato, corn and other grains, soya, salt and sugar. These are the building blocks of industrial food. They are moulded, shaped, puffed and strung into every shape and texture you can imagine so that their raw identities become obscure and unknowable. Very clever food engineering may be great for mouth-feel, but is it mouth-real? One of the joys of dining is the knowledge that you, or someone close to you, has created a genuine meal, poured something of themselves into it and not just heated up some gloop.

If you have not cooked much before, then I say to you 'fear not'. Start with something easy to succeed at, like a Niçoise salad (quick, easy, delicious) or a chicken stir-fry. There is a wealth of advice out there on the internet for the novice. Two of my favourites are Facebook's 'Let's Get Banting UK' group and dietdoctor.com. Oh and do not forget to watch the film *Julie and Julia* for some fantasy culinary inspiration. Another thing worth mentioning about cooking is that it is a good idea to build up a repertoire of, say, ten or a dozen dishes that you prepare regularly. You will get better at consistently producing low-carb meals that are great with regular practice; cultivate those micro-skills. My regulars list includes things like a variety of easy-to-assemble salads, griddled salmon steaks with pesto, Spanish pork stew with chorizo, all-day breakfast (but cooked for supper) and... well, it's over to you now.

Michael Pollan, the renowned American investigative journalist, described trying out various eating styles for his book *The Omnivore's Dilemma*[1]. He later covered the same ground in his film *Food, Inc.*[2] Pollan foraged hunter-gatherer fashion in California. He ate the organic way too, but he also described trying out what average Americans now commonly eat. Not surprisingly, he found that cheap food comes at the expense of farm workers' happiness, factory worker's rights, animal welfare, consumer value and the nation's health. Shockingly, the whole agri-business merry-go-round is subsidised by the taxpayer. American citizens actually subsidise production of the very junk food that is making them so overweight and ill and it is rapidly bankrupting their health services (and increasingly so in the UK too).

One statistic Pollan gave was particularly mind-boggling. At the time of writing in 2006, he reported that one in five meals in America was consumed in a motor vehicle. So, for this part of his gastronomic journey, Pollan and his family dutifully ate their 14-dollar's worth of burgers, nuggets, fries and cobb salad washed down with a cola drink while driving at 55mph over the Golden Gate Bridge from Marin County south to San Francisco. A point he has made more than once in his writing is that there is a world of difference between eating and dining. We all have to eat but if there were to be a reworking of the Ten Commandments, for me one of them would be 'Thou shalt Dine'. Healthy eating for those with diabetes or pre-diabetes demands not just that food is low-carb but that the time, place and ambience are right too. Thou must dine.

So, what is the difference between eating and dining? Perhaps it is easier to say what dining actually is. Dining, in my book, is the sociable sharing of food that has been presented as a meal. It is more than just an exercise in refuelling. It is usually but not necessarily a social activity. Dining is an occasion. We often gather together to dine. We usually dine at a table, which may have been prepared to both complement and enhance the meal to be consumed. Pollan contends that 'a desk is not a table'. Dining requires respect for the food as well as the cook. Dining should be unhurried: dining is usually 'slow food'. You may enjoy conversation as you dine but keep it face-to-face with your fellow diners. Shun that smart phone during meals and ditch that tablet too. When at the table be 100% present in the culinary and social moment.

I have come across some who suggested we should not eat any food that can be consumed standing up; rather prefer food for which a table is essential. I would not go that far, but I would agree that eating on the go can be dangerous. Consuming food while not seated at a table runs the risk of mindless eating and chomping on autopilot. It is of necessity quick eating and that risks over-eating; by the time our stomach says 'enough, put the food down and come out with your hands up', it is too late. Satiety (feeling full-up) signals just don't kick in quickly enough when we eat rapidly. The bottom lines are dine at a table, eat slowly and stop eating before you are full.

How different this is from what has come to be commonplace these days. We now seem content to eat on our laps in front of the telly, or walking down the street, or reading a magazine, or checking out social media. Eating has also become an integral part of what were previously considered non-eating activities. Why for example do we feel it necessary to munch through a bucket of popcorn at the cinema? Is it really possible to fully enjoy the chomped popcorn and properly appreciate a film at the same time? Why do we now think it just fine to eat tray-loads of chips, or worse still, those horrid unspecified meat (presumably mammal-based) burgers and pies when attending football matches, just an hour or two after having eaten lunch? This is not about nourishment; it is behaviour and mindlessly bad behaviour at that.

Yes, eating, like so many of the activities we engage in, is a manifestation of behaviour. It is something we do. Sometimes it is deliberately learned behaviour, but as often as not it has just been absorbed silently and become an un-thought-through default habit. As we grow up, we observe, usually subconsciously, what goes on around us. This automatically sinks into our brains and becomes our normality. The world we inhabit is normal for us, no matter how odd it might appear to an outsider. Actually, you could say it is only normal in a mathematical sense, i.e. average behaviour within a population. Is it truly humanly normal to eat mindlessly? Certainly, it cannot be considered dining.

Mindless eating, now the norm, has its dangers. Consuming that presumably mammal-based-meat pie with a portion of chips at the football match, or a bucket of popcorn while watching a film, surely means we are not engaging in either activity properly? Because the types of food consumed on autopilot are almost always cheap, carbohydrate-dense, heavily processed industrial offerings, it allows us to eat far more than we might otherwise have done had we sat down at a table in the company of friends. Mindless eating is the opposite of dining because, not only is mindlessly eaten food typically low quality, Big-6 heavy and stuffed with ingredients best avoided, it so often fails to satisfy our appetites for long either. Perhaps it is only tolerable to eat such fodder when distracted; had we permitted our attention to focus on it clearly, we may have felt revolted.

So, do not eat on the go, or working at a desk, or playing a computer game, or watching a film, or reading this book. Instead dine and when you eat ensure it is an enjoyable experience. It is possible to both dine alone and dine on food that can be prepared in a few seconds; how about a slice of ham with pickles and a few lettuce leaves, splashed with vinaigrette dressing? Have a couple of wedges of cheese too, if you are still peckish. It is possible to dine without a table; picnics for example. It is even possible to dine on a seaside bench on fish and chips from a newspaper wrap (occasionally). Perhaps dining is an attitude, a frame of mind. Dining involves concentration on, indulgence in and enjoyment of real food. So, be mindful with that meal.

Did I just say fish and chips? Indeed I did, for even chips are not under an absolute ban. Nothing is. Eat and drink merrily anything you want, more or less. I might draw the line at sweetened fizzy drinks (unless I was clinically dehydrated and no other treatment was available) or tripe (because it really does not appeal to me) and, of course, trans-fats but otherwise eat whatever you want. The crucial thing about eating items from the Out-Foods list is that it boils down to how much and how often you eat them. So, I will happily eat fish 'n chips, with plenty of salt and vinegar. When I go back to the Greystones Road chip shop in sunny Sheffield, I will enjoy them with a bread cake too. I will only eat them once or perhaps twice a year. Fish 'n chips is an occasional treat; a feast. It does not and never will, form part of my usual regular staple diet. When I eat them, I make sure I thoroughly enjoy them. They are too naughty to be consumed mindlessly. So, whether they come wrapped from the Greystones chippie to be eaten at home, or enjoyed 'open' straight from the paper on Aldeburgh Beach, I concentrate on the taste and I do so in company. I have even been known to eat fish 'n chips in a car but only when parked up. Actually, it was raining at the time.

As St. Paul the Apostle said, *The strength of sin is the law* [3]. Laws always seem to have escape clauses that can be manipulated by the devious, the weak willed and, of course, lawyers. So, again I say, stick with the principles of the *Beating Diabetes* approach and adhere to the spirit of the law rather than the word.

This same advice goes for each and every other item on the Out-Foods list. So, when in France, bag a baguette. When in New York, fill your belly in a deli. When in Delhi, have a chapatti with your curry. It is all about distinguishing staple foods from the occasional off-piste feast.

Practical suggestions

- **If you have a significant other, be honest them.** Consider two scenarios. In one, both the person with diabetes and their partner think trying out a different style of eating and dining would be a great idea. They will, no doubt, keep on reading with a positive outlook and probably anticipate with mounting excitement the different meals they are about to try. Feel their enthusiasm. In the other scenario, both parties think that diet change is neither desirable nor practical. They too will move forward in unison. All they need to do is decide what happens to this flipping book but there are two other possible scenarios. Maybe the person with diabetes wishes to institute change but their significant other is less than keen. Or how about if the diabetic person's partner is of the opinion that diet change is what is needed but the poor old victim is less than enthusiastic? Oh dear, very choppy waters. Running two menus in parallel is an option but stormy weather lies ahead in their kitchen. The point is, this needs to be discussed openly before rushing headlong into low-carb dining to the dismay of the other person. Parallel cooking is possible. Mother may still have potato with her roast chicken, or toast for breakfast and father might have steamed vegetables and boiled eggs instead. Better to jaw-jaw than war-war over the dining table.
- **Work out a meal plan:** I know of some folk who roll the same plan through every week. It is Tuesday so must be salmon and pesto, for example. Groundhog Week dining. A rolling plan might be fine or you may prefer some variety. Decide what will work for you. Obviously, events and other commitments will intrude at times, so flexibility is important. The beauty of a meal plan is that it avoids the desperate 5pm 'what shall we have for dinner tonight, darling?' head-scratch. Once you have planned a few meals (and do make sure some will leave enough left overs to feed into the next day's meals as well. For example, Spanish style pork stew or

roast chicken), then you can move on to drawing up a list. I have posted a 7-day, 3-meals-a-day plan below (Table 5.1).

- **The joy of lists:** I would be sunk without a list when I go to shop. At my age, I find keeping four or more items in mind hard enough, let alone a full shopping manifest. So, get listing. That way you will shop smarter, quicker and more cheaply. You will be less tempted to be called into the deepest recesses of the processed and packaged food aisles of the supermarket too. It you always work from a list and something is missing, then it is not your fault. 'Well, if it wasn't on the list...'

- **Plan that shopping trip:** They say never go food shopping when you are hungry. It is a risky business stepping out of your door and placing yourself in temptation's way. This is one situation where a small appetite-busting snack beforehand might actually be a good idea. A friend told me to make sure and take my glasses with me. That way I will be able to read the small print about what is actually in the product I am considering buying. You can bet that if 'low-fat' is plastered all over the container in lurid colours, there will also be a small table, covered in microscopic writing hidden on the side or back, revealing the less palatable truth about its high-carb credentials. Of course, do not forget to take that list with you.

- **And clear those cupboards:** A tricky one this. No one likes waste. Getting rid of jars of jam or packets of frosted breakfast flakes feels wrong in one way but consider this, if you are going low-carb, do you really want these food items hanging around like little bits of unexploded ordnance, just waiting to blow your resolve into bits? No, of course not. So, sweep through those cupboards and pantries and purge them of their Out-Food contents. You know it makes sense.

- **And finally, remember you are low-carb dining**: What you are not doing is a low-calorie thing. If you cut the cals, you risk sliding into starvation mode, a mode where metabolism slows and the need for calories drops. Low-cal is a diminishing-returns strategy. It is a moving goalpost trap; that is why it so often fails and that is why it is to be avoided. So, good news. As long as you keep the sugary and starchy carbs low, you do not need to fret so much about the quantity of food you eat when it comes to dining. Low-carb is almost always a higher-fat approach and fat is not just tasty, it is satisfying – it fills you up; it flicks the full-up switch better and for longer far than carbs. Fat has the satiety factor. Now isn't that a lovely thought?

A word or two about danger meals

- **Eating out:** Suddenly you have lost control. An item of food like, for example a dressed salad, which at home would be a delightful low-carb creation, suddenly becomes a biohazard. Out there, in Fast-Food Diner-land, it may have croutons, small gobbets of pure starch fried in a cheap Omega-6 heavy oil. It may have a commercial dressing tipped over it too, which in all likelihood will be sweetened with sugar and thickened with starch. That salad may come in with a calorie ticket higher than the burger and fries you may have thought was the less healthy option. Or how about a lunch that starts with bread rolls on a side plate, followed by a choice of rice, fries or couscous with the main course? You need to consider your dietary rules of engagement before you leave your house. Could you take a small container of homemade vinaigrette to dress a plain salad with you? Might you delay meeting up with your friends until after they have chomped through their fast food? You could excuse yourself with 'actually, I have already eaten, so perhaps just a diet cola, a cup of coffee, or the cheese board.' Be prepared.
- **Festive feasts:** 'But we always have parsnips, roast potatoes and bread sauce with turkey at Christmas, Thanksgiving or Grandad's birthday. What is wrong with you?' Tricky. Again, plan and be prepared. Tell the host in advance you have a medical condition and that your doctor has put you on a restricted diet. Hey! I am a

doctor. Tell them I told you. The possibilities for straying into high-carb territory are endless, particularly for some of those westernised versions of Asian and Oriental food with their special rice, battered items and sweet sticky sauces.

- **Corporate conundrums featuring Buffet the diabetes slayer**: Most help-yourself buffets, whether at birthday celebrations or bar mitzvahs, wakes or welcomes are almost always a double whammy of a problem. Firstly, when faced with a selection, we humans have an almost irresistible urge to try out a bit of everything. Your brain will already be motoring into its default over-eating mode before you confront problem number 2: buffets. Buffets are almost always sugary and starchy to the exclusion of almost anything else. Buffets are almost always a carb-ageddon, affair in beige, temptingly presented on a long table. Always beware beige foods like open sandwiches, closed sandwiches, crusty quiches, pies, baked potatoes, floury wraps, breaded onion rings, scotch eggs, sausage rolls or crisps. The only apparently less un-healthy choices are likely to be fruity offerings and sugary yoghurts. So why not just tell yourself that you do not depend on the buffet for your nutritional wellbeing? Indulging in the wrong stuff when you are not malnourished or dying of starvation is a manifestation of weak or thoughtless behaviour. Think about it beforehand. Say to yourself and your hosts that you have already eaten. Even better, why not actually eat something beforehand? Do not let yourself slide into a disaster. Okay, so we all lapse occasionally but, as Maria Platts, a research nurse colleague in Sheffield once said, "Don't let your lapses become relapses".
- **Death by dinner party:** This scenario is a mash-up of the festive and the corporate buffet ambush and should be countered with the same strategies. Tell them your doctor has put you on a strict exclusion diet. Blame me again if you like. Or offer to bring something yourself to spare your host a headache and you the embarrassment. Failing that, accept small portions and

leave what you do not wish to eat. The hazards are legion as will be the solutions. Just keep your eyes and mind open and deploy your strategies with forethought.

A word about snacks

Precisely the same principle applies to eating snacks between meals. *Shop, Cook, Dine* (if possible) and enjoy but if you are a secret snacker, make sure that, if you absolutely must graze, do so *glucose-insulin-lite*. Snacks, like regular meals, do need some planning. Basically, ask yourself whether snacks should be prepared in advance, standing by ready to be consumed. I think the answer to that is usually yes. So again, be prepared; get one jump ahead; add them to your list. If you go hunting for food when the hunger urge hits you, you are more likely to gather a plate full of all the Out-Foods you can find and that is not good. The same thing happens when we feel peckish between meals. If you go on the snack hunt with no *on-piste* options easily available, you are courting trouble.

If you must have one, the ideal snack should be *glucose-insulin-lite* and yet filling enough to quell the appetite until the next proper meal comes around. How about carrot sticks and hummus, or an egg you boiled earlier, or some nibbles of cheese? Or perhaps a few nuts but not a round of sandwiches, or a packet of cheesy you-know-whatsits. Get the right stuff in and keep it handy.

Having said that, there is a significant down side to snacking and it is to do with its effects on body chemistry. I am not a believer in frequent small meals; they just keep food-derived glucose tickling away at our insulin response non-stop and without respite. Any food consumed between meals breaks the period of fasting and fasting is a good thing, even those brief fasts between lunch and supper. Perhaps the most dangerous snack is the one most loved by Hobbits: the after-supper morsel[4]. These late-night snacks delay the start of the circadian overnight switch from burning meal-derived sugar to liver-derived glycogen-sugar and beyond into fat (more about the joy of fasting later). So, *Beating Diabetes* says avoid snacking, especially and particularly late at night, but if you must nibble, prepare ahead – mitigate those morsels.

A little afterthought: food is not a reward

Eating is a manifestation of behaviour. Sometimes eating is about nutrition, but too often it degenerates into something we just do, like the horrid mammal-pie wolfed down outside the football ground, or in my case the rubbish hotdog reward for enduring another boring circuit around a certain Scandinavian furniture warehouse with the missus. I suppose special meals, feasts, parties, fish 'n chips on Aldeburgh beach can also be rewarding. We all, at times, use food as tokens of reward for work done or traumas suffered but when this spills over into everyday life, we get into trouble.

I have had one hell of a morning, so I deserve some biscuits.
I have kept to the diet for a week, so tomorrow I will wallow in chocolate.
You looked after me so well. Here is some cake.

This displaces food from the dining table into a sneaky dark corner of our life and we don't just do it to ourselves, we do it to others too, particularly our kids.
You have been a very good little girl. Have some sweets.
You have been a naughty little boy. No sweets for you!

Reward-food is almost always off-piste fodder, stuff from the Out-Foods list. I do not mean to be a killjoy, rather I would just like to shine a little light into that murky area deep in our psyches. Know food rewards for what they are – trouble, in more ways than one. Sermon over.

Conclusion

In the next chapter, we will explore the amazing world of intermittent fasting. A fascinating topic and not nearly as scary as you might think. Fasting is something we can deploy and use very much to our metabolic advantage. Yes, fasting can be painless, fun even; and it can turbo-charge dietary change.

Notes:

1. The Omnivore's Dilemma: A Natural History Of Four Meals. Michael Pollan. Published by PublicAffairs.
2. See also his DVD 'Food, Inc.: How industrial food is making us sicker, fatter and poorer – and what you can do about it'. *https://www.imdb.com/title/tt1286537/.*
3. *The sting of death is sin and the strength of sin is the law* (1 r 15 v 56 NKJV).
4. The after-supper morsel was the last meal of the day for Hobbits. Bilbo Baggins had saved two seed cakes for his after-supper enjoyment before he was rudely interrupted in *An Unexpected Party*. We of course are not hobbits who presumably had more robust metabolisms. The Hobbit. Published by Allen and Unwin.

Table 5.1 – A specimen 7-day meal plan

	Breakfast *	Light meal	Main meal
Sunday	Poached egg on spinach	Cheese, ham, pickle ploughman's	Roast chicken **, with green beans and steamed broccoli, Coconut yoghurt ice cream
Monday	2 boiled eggs	Chicken mayo salad	Baked salmon and pesto with green beans and steamed broccoli, Blueberries and cream
Tuesday	Greek yoghurt with blueberries	Flaked leftover salmon with mayo on an avocado green salad	Onion soup with chicken stock, fried haloumis bacon wraps on green salad, Chocolate mousse
Wednesday	2 sausages with mushrooms	Leftover onion soup	Egg and avocado mayo with green salad, Strawberries and cream
Thursday	Scrambled eggs with smoked salmon topping	Cheese, ham, pickle ploughman's	Spanish pork stew, green salad, Nut-granola on ice cream
Friday	Home-made nut-granola *** on Greek yoghurt	Leftover pork stew	Courgetti with kale, feta and pesto, Tiramisu
Saturday	Full English: egg, bacon, black pudding with fried tomatoes	Almond flour based mini pizzas	Tuna Niçoise salad, Coconut yoghurt ice cream

Note: In any seven-day period I generally aim for:

- 2 Meat/poultry dishes
- 2 Fish dishes
- 2 Vegetarian dishes
- +1 other choice

* You do not have to eat breakfast if you prefer not to. You can instead extend your overnight fast until lunchtime. See the chapter on Fasting for details. More often than not I now breakfast late and have nothing to eat until dinner; my second and final meal of the day

Chapter 6 – Fast

Oh, the delight that is fasting. It really is up there with writing lists but I can only imagine the horror that you may be feeling right now. Fasting does sound bad, doesn't it? Actually, fasting comes in many shapes and forms, so if you like, why not consider picking one that suits you. You could even mix and match with two types if you want. You may be interested to know that simply combining an early evening meal with a late breakfast the next day is perhaps the most basic form of fasting. By stretching your natural overnight fast at both ends, you can slide you painlessly into an insulin-free fat-burning mode.

Fasting has a very long and worthy history in religion. Christians traditionally fasted through Advent in the run up to Christmas and of course during the six weeks of Lent before Easter. Muslims famously fast observantly during daylight hours through the holy month of Ramadan. Many Jews fast on Rosh Hashanah. Buddhists may fast to improve awareness during meditation, or as a spiritual discipline. Hindus often fast from midnight through to midday, which, as we shall see, is one of the fasting options that may help with diabetes. For Sikhs, however, religious fasting appears to have been prohibited by the Sri Guru Granth Sahib but only as an idolatrous practice. Health motivated fasts may, I suspect, be allowed. The big question for most people is 'why bother?' What has fasting ever done for us?

To answer that question, we are going to have to dive back into the workings of the human body once more and discover what a wonderful multi-fuel-powered machine it is. So again, apologies in advance if there is some technical detail to get your head around. As before, may I commend it to you? When you know how your body is powered, you will be rewarded with some very useful insights and the ability to choose between one fuel option and another. If you cannot wait to get to the nuts and bolts of fasting you could skip the Power to the people section; but you will be missing out.

In this chapter I will use the scientifically correct term 'glucose' rather than previously where I have used the generic term sugar. I have done this for precision and clarity.

Power to the people

Ask most people and this includes most health professionals, what powers the body, what keeps the show on the road and the answer will be 'food'. Ask those same people if there is any other source of energy the body can use and they may vaguely say 'our body fat stores'. Both answers are, of course, correct, but only as far as they go. A little more understanding of the ways our bodies keep the heart pumping and the brain thinking can be truly enlightening and particularly useful for weight loss and regaining control of diabetes. This is because it reveals why so many of us get fat and diabetic in the first place and, importantly, how smart-fasting may boost the low carb approach's benefits. Understanding this will enable you to choose which power source you want to run on and precisely when it is best for you to do it. It isn't difficult, but it is a powerful tool that can in correcting the devastating effects of our modern carb-dominated diet.

Basically, there are three healthy fuel options open to the body. Firstly, every time we eat, we absorb nutrients during digestion to power our body's engines. Secondly, between meals, we switch seamlessly over to our reserve sugar stash, glycogen. Then, if we have not eaten for a while and all the glycogen has gone, we seamlessly switch over to our third fuel option, we start burning our fat. Man (and woman) can live by fat alone. Let's look at food glucose, glycogen glucose and our fat-burning modes in a little more depth. A knowledge of each will allow you to know about and even choose which fuel mode you desire to use.

1 - **Food.** It is obvious, isn't it? We need to eat to live. Food brings us carbs, fats and proteins in various combinations. It also gives us minerals, vitamins and fibre but, more than that, food can be the source of enormous blessing and pleasure. When considering how to prevent or treat diabetes, we really need to focus on sugary and starchy carbs, the ones that push blood glucose (sugar) levels up during digestion.

Imagine eating a high-carb snack or meal. Your body will use the glucose it gets for any immediate energy needs, like walking up a flight of stairs, pumping blood around, or even reading this book perhaps. Secondly, if necessary, it will top up your glycogen stores (this is called glycogenesis – making glycogen from glucose). Meeting immediate energy needs and replenishing glycogen stores are 'insulin-sparing' and they happen pretty much on their own. After that, all the remaining glucose in the bloodstream has to be cleared away and that is when insulin does its thing. Insulin converts all the excess glucose into fat (this is called lipogenesis – making fat from glucose). Insulin then pushes the newly formed fats it into your fat cells. None of this is contentious and none of this should come as a shock. Insulin is, after, all our hormone of energy storage; and it with deals any surplus glucose-energy very efficiently. Usually, by around two hours after you have finished that carby meal, all the glucose will have been cleared form the blood stream (unless you are diabetic or pre-diabetic).

2 - Glycogen. Okay, so it is now a couple of hours after you ate that carby meal, your blood glucose surge has been sorted out. Insulin has brought things back into balance. Good old insulin. Then what? Will you go all wobbly? Will your blood glucose levels continue dropping until topped up by the next carby meal? Well, no. That is because you have a carbohydrate store inside your body. You just switch over to burning those reserves instead. That reserve carb store, sitting there waiting for you to draw on it, is something called glycogen, which we keep in the liver (See Figure 6.1). Glycogen is a glucose polymer. Yup, it is a form of starch. Actually, there is glycogen in your muscles too, quite a lot of it, but muscles tend to hang on to it. They don't contribute much to maintaining blood glucose levels. Liver glycogen is the stuff you use between meals to keep your glucose levels up in the normal healthy range and glycogen comes into its own every single night. Your tissues and organs extract glucose all the time, even when you are asleep. So, when your blood levels start to dip, your liver obligingly breaks down some glycogen and quietly trickles glucose back into your bloodstream, while you sleep (this is called glycogenolysis – glycogen breakdown to make glucose). You may be asleep, but your blood glucose level needs topping up constantly. It is used to keep you warm and breathing and perhaps even dreaming too. Your stock of liver glycogen can keep things going for around twelve hours. So, if you dine at 8pm, your food derived blood glucose will clear over the next couple of hours and by 10.00-10.30pm, glycogen will start to kick in. You will flip from clearing glucose away to trickling it back into the circulation.

If you rise and breakfast at 8am the next day, you will not have run out of glycogen, although the tank will be running low. If however, you miss breakfast and your natural overnight fast is stretched longer than twelve hours, or if during this time you undertake significant physical exercise, you will run out of glycogen. Then what? Will you go all wobbly? Will your blood glucose levels drop at that point? Well no. Again, you won't just keel over and die. That is because when there is no food-derived glucose left and your glycogen/glucose stores have run dry and another of your body's natural power sources kicks in, fat (see Figure 6.1 again). Actually, you will still need to keep your glucose levels stable. So, if necessary, proteins in the body can be transformed into glucose and you won't need much because, by then, most of your energy needs will be supplied from fat alone.

3 - Fat. It is obvious really. Like many of the body's systems, blood glucose levels are closely controlled. Its levels are kept strictly within a very tight range, never allowed to go too low and never too high, assuming you are healthy that is. If glucose drifts up, insulin brings it down and if it drifts down, other hormones like glucagon bring it up. When all the glycogen has been burned, it is our fat stores that get tapped into next. Fat is, after all, just stored energy. Weight for weight, it stores over twice the energy of proteins and carbohydrates. Fat is 'calorie-dense'. Fat cannot be transformed back into glucose in any meaningful quantity. When we use our fat stores to provide energy, it is fatty acids that get released into the circulation (lipolysis). If we need glucose when we are fasting, we get it from protein (gluconeogenesis – making glucose from something else, like protein). Of course, if we eat any protein-containing food, it will spare our body-proteins from being burned, which is good. Body-proteins include things like our muscles. Short fasts make virtually no difference to body protein levels, whereas prolonged calorie restriction (starvation) certainly does. Anyway, burning fat/fatty acids is good and is, in fact, what a lot of us need to do. That is because burning fat is also known as losing weight. You cannot switch over to your fat-burning mode if glucose is being fed into the bloodstream from your food or drink, or from your liver-glycogen.

Actually, there is another fat-burning mode. Our bodies can motor along burning fat but fatty acids cannot be used to fuel the brain. For that we need glucose or another type of fuel called ketones and your body can happily make ketones from fatty acids in your liver.

Like the word diabetes, ketosis is another with more than one meaning. Diabetic ketosis, also known as keto-acidosis, is a severe complication of Type-1 Diabetes (and also as a complication with some of the drugs given in Type-2 Diabetes). It needs urgent medical treatment if coma and death are to be avoided. It is a dangerous and abnormal chemical derangement. Dietary ketosis on the other hand sounds the same but it isn't. It is a totally different thing. It is a benign, natural, normal and positively healthful thing. Ketosis was probably the main energy mode that kept humanity going for its first 230,000 years tramping across this planet; before farming gifted us sugary and starchy carbs and insulin excess suddenly became a very necessary compensation for our new normal state of affairs. There is a whole keto-world out there on the net.

Keto-dieting may seem extreme but many chose it as a form of healthy eating that are almost totally free of sugars and starches. It isn't something I do personally, but you may well come across information about it if you search the net. The aim of very low or even zero-carb eating is to deliberately switch the body over to its fat-burning-ketosis mode permanently. The amount of protein foods may also have to be watched to get into ketosis. These 'ketotic' or 'keto-adapted' diets are not as whacky as you may imagine. In fact, ketosis diets are a well-recognised treatment used by doctors to help people with intractable epilepsy, particularly children. They can be highly effective in reducing the frequency and severity of seizures. Ketosis diets are generally used when medication has failed to control things acceptably. There is also evidence that keto-diets may be beneficial in people with a variety of cancers, including brain cancer. It appears that some cancer cells are particularly dependent on glucose for their energy needs. When deprived of glucose and served with ketones instead, the balance between progression and remission of the tumour can improve. Normal cells like using ketones. Cancer cells sometimes don't. For me personally, though, for the present at least, I would find a full-on ketosis diet a hardship; I'm a lowish-carb, not a no-carb, person. That is not to say that it isn't a good diet to follow. By the way, you may not be surprised to learn that funding for trials of keto-diets in cancer for example, unlike developing sexy novel and potentially profitable drugs, is rare. See *Fail* for further discussion of very low-carb diets.

So now you know. If you choose to have frequent small sugary or starchy meals like the ones most Official guidelines recommend, you will inevitably have a food-glucose/insulin dominated body chemistry. If the sugary tap is never turned off you will never be free of insulin domination. Your biology will have no choice but to work this way. If you eat like this all the time, you are putting yourself at risk of both weight gain and Type-2 Diabetes, as well as a fatty liver and fatty pancreas. If you already have diabetes and follow Official advice and feast frequently on carbs, you will likely need to take drugs to treat the consequences of those food choices.

On the other hand, if you choose to have well-spaced out low-carb meals and refrain from snacking in between, you will be much more likely to use your own fat stores for fuel, which is to say you will lose weight. You will be less likely to develop insulin resistance, which is to say, develop diabetes. If you choose to time your eating patterns wisely in ways that allow fat burning to kick in, you are likely restore a normal body chemistry. In short, you will keep insulin levels as nature intended them to be – minimal. So, that is the low down on how our bodies and wonderful multi-fuel machines but what about fasting and exercise?

Figure 6.1 The four principal fuel sources that power the body

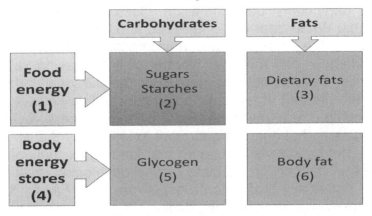

Figure 6.1 The fuels our bodies are principally adapted to use are carbohydrates and fats. These can be obtained from food of course but they can also be obtained from the body's internal carbohydrate and fat stores. Knowing that we are multi-fuel machines can allow us to deliberately choose which fuel to run on.

1. So, food obviously. We need to eat certain (so called essential) fats and proteins to maintain a healthy body but we also eat carbs, fats and proteins to provide us with energy

116

2. Sugary and starchy foods are the potent carbohydrates that liberate glucose. Our bodies need glucose and one way to get it (but not the only way) is to eat carbohydrate containing foods and it is these food-derived sugars and starches that together drive many into Type-2 diabetes
3. Fats derived from a variety of foods can also be used to 'burn' as fuel. However, if there is any surplus glucose around and when insulin is being secreted, fat will not be used as fuel. It will be stored. If you want to use food derived fat for power you can only do so if starchy and sugary foods are avoided. When carbs/glucose/insulin is around dietary fats will be sent straight to storage
4. We have energy stored up in our bodies. It's like switching over to battery power when the food energy has been used. These energy stores allow us to survive between meals and overnight and early on during periods of fasting
5. The first battery we tap into between meals is glycogen. Our liver has enough of the stuff to keep us going for 12-16 hours. The switch to glycogen 'burning' happens automatically when food derived glucose is cleared from the blood stream
6. When the glycogen store is empty up we make another automatic fuel-switch. Our second battery power source comes on-line; we start burning body fat. Around 16-20 hours after we consumed our last meal we start to rely on fat for power. Burning body fat is good for weight loss (obviously). People who eat minimal or no carbs function purely on power from fat, either derived from food or from the body's fat stores

Actually, there are two other fuel sources that you should know about. Protein from food can be chemically converted to make glucose and, during starvation, body proteins e.g. muscle tissue) can be used to make fuel. The other is alcohol, which is a sort of carbohydrate. Although it does not produce glucose, it can be used to generate energy.

Fasting

Until recently, at Christmas usually, someone from the British Dietetic Association (BDA) posted a semi-jokey article online for their reader's amusement about the year's top Celeb Diets. I am not sure who reads it other than other dieticians and me. Anyway, you could read it on their website. And every year, some form of low-carb diet or some form of Intermittent Fasting diet, or both, used to make it to their top 5. The BDA loved to give these approaches a bit of a kicking each year, and when better than Christmas? 'Tis the season to be contrary. It seems this year (2019) they have gone strangely quiet on low-carb and fasting. Is appeasement in the air?

The BDA previously did this, I assume, because those diets challenge both their orthodox beliefs and their authority in matters to do with diets. Dieticians surely should be the ones in charge of all things nutritional. Just as doctors seem to own diseases, dieticians own diets, or at least some seem to behave as if they do. For most, their belief is in adhering to a "balanced diet", a diet based firmly on two things. Firstly, the benefits of eating plenty of "healthy" carbs, like potatoes, fruit, and wholegrain cereals plus vegetables. They dislike adding sugars (extrinsic sugars) to food and drinks (good) but do not object to, in fact they actively promote, consuming carby foods and drinks that naturally evoke significant sugar surges into the bloodstream (not so good; and, in my opinion, bad). To them, therefore, a low-carb diet must be wrong, a heresy that deserves to be stamped on with great vigour. After all, low-carb means no baked potatoes with baked beans, or spaghetti. In fact, in a number of countries around the world (Australia and South Africa in particular), dieticians who have lost the faith, and other health professionals, who promote low-carb diet approaches, have been subjected to harsh and intense litigation, disciplinary proceedings and threatened with removal of their licence to practice. Professionally 'game-over', in other words.

Secondly, the BDA (at the time of writing) adheres to the calories-in/calories out-theory. It underlies their understanding of how a healthy weight is maintained. Calorie-control is, in their view, a zero-sum thing, it is a form of energy accountancy, and fasting is, in their view, just another faddish way of eating fewer calories. And worse, fasting has become an even more significant fad since the health journalist and broadcaster Dr. Michael Mosely investigated it in a programme, which was shown in the UK and worldwide on BBC TV (1). Even worse, Mosley's programme was followed by a hugely successful book co-written with Mimi Spencer – *The Fast Diet*.[2]

For the BDA, intermittent fasting is just another stupid diet fad, something to laugh at; something to ridicule. But curiously, huge numbers of people who have tried it for themselves have found that it can work, and work well. You can lose weight by fasting periodically. A quick disclaimer here. I am not advising anyone to undertake Intermittent Fasting. In fact, I think switching to a low-carb *Beating Diabetes* eating regime alone would benefit the health of most people who currently adhere to Official diet guidelines. It is up to you, but read on to discover what it is all about, and why I believe Intermittent Fasting has significant potential benefits, why it may turbo-charge the low-carb approach.

So, what is Intermittent Fasting? Is it just a fancy way of cutting calories, or is it doing something completely different? Well, you are now familiar with the various options the body has at its disposal to keep us constantly supplied with energy. Eating is the most common method, obviously, but, as you can see, we can function between meals quite nicely without consuming any food at all. Mosely and Spencer's fasting method isn't actually a total fast at all. They simply advise that, for two days each week, followers cut their food calorie intake down to around 500 for women, 600 for men. They do not even advise whether those calories should be low-carb or not, nor whether they should be consumed in one, two or even three meals across the fast-day. Because for the other five days of the week followers can eat normally, their method is called the 5:2 Diet. I have encountered many people, family members included, who have discovered it for themselves.

They just started practicing the 5:2 approach off their own bat, without permission from their dieticians or doctors, and found it a pretty painless way to lose weight. In fact, because it is a diet that the Official guidelines and legions of health professionals neither promote nor advise, I call it a *people's diet*. 5:2-ers, it seems, know something that many of their doctors and dieticians do not.

The 5:2 and other similar diets may result in a small reduction in calorie intake, but over the week as a whole the absolute calorie reduction is minimal. In my view it works not because it induces a "calorie deficit" but rather because it switches the body's energy supply from the food-glucose mode, through glycogen and into its fat burning modes. It therefore reliably reduces insulin production and allows, for a day or two each week at least, one's body chemistry to recover. It is about body chemistry, not calorie accountancy. Remember, it is difficult to store fat in the absence of insulin, and you cannot lose fat in its presence.

I tried the 5:2 myself once and I was quite pleased with the result. It did help me to lose some weight, even though my overall weekly calorie intake didn't change much. I ate a little more on post-fast days, I suppose. I chose to do my fasts on busy days. I figured that being busy would distract me from my stomach's grumblings, which in fact, it did. Eventually, however, I found that my will power became a problem and I stopped. Fasting during the day was not an issue, but when I got back home for my evening meal, I lapsed. Most people, it seems, are stronger willed than I (*mea culpa*) and have learned to celebrate those brief sensations of hunger for what they are: a sign of the body switching over to fat burning.

There are many other ways to fast. Currently I have found another one that suits me much better. Like those Hindu fasters mentioned earlier, I simply skip breakfast most days. I try to eat my evening meal the night before as early as I can (usually around 8pm although earlier still would be better – *mea maxima culpa*). I particularly choose low-carb ingredients for that meal then eat nothing until noon the next day, or sometimes later. I guess it regularly leaves me food-glucose free for around 16 hours at a stretch. This seems to work for me and is a method I find very easy to apply. My understanding of its mechanism (how it works, in other words) is that the evening meal does not evoke much of a glucose-insulin response. This allows me to enter my natural overnight glycogen-burning mode before I even go to bed. Then, sometime around dawn, when my glycogen tank runs out, I switch over to fat burning. I carry on fat burning after I rise through until I break my fast around noon or 1pm. I will drink during this time and have water, tea or coffee with a dash of milk (a small carb dose here), but it works. It is a short absolute fast rather than a longer relative one like the 5:2 diet, but, like the 5:2, it is Intermittent. I can eat normally when I am not fasting. I am not on a starvation programme.

More demanding fasting regimes might include ones where followers have a partial or total fast every other day; not something for weak-willed people like me. Another is known as the 8-Hour Diet. (See Table 6.2 for a bird's-eye view of various fasting options). It requires its followers to eat all their meals within an eight-hour period, between 10am and 6pm say, or 12 noon and 8pm, for example. For the other sixteen hours they eat nothing but may drink water. This is also called "restricted eating" and it is, more or less, my current habit. But all these fasts all end up doing just one thing to a greater or lesser extent. They switch insulin off, and turn the fat burning mode on.

The one thing that modern fasting isn't is starvation. Fasting switches fuel sources around allowing insulin levels to drop and fat to be mobilised. Although these changes also occur during starvation several other less desirable adaptations to severe food restriction happen as well. Firstly, the body senses it is entering a starvation state and starts to economise. It will slow down its metabolic rate causing lethargy and a feeling of cold. Secondly, it diverts its conscious priorities towards food seeking. People become obsessed about food and it will occupy their thoughts intrusively. And thirdly, if sugary, starchy and protein foods are limited during starvation the body begins to convert some of its own proteins into glucose causing a loss of muscle mass. Fat cannot be converted back into glucose in any meaningful amounts. Starving people will waste away. Those who fast do not experience these drastic starvation-type effects because their dietary protein intake will be sufficient to produce glucose without the need to degrade muscle tissue, even if they do not consume any carbs at all.

Is this relevant to *Beating Diabetes*? The answer is yes, because a form of starvation therapy is currently advocated as a means of putting diabetes into remission. It is called very low-calorie (VLC) food replacement therapy. This involves cutting daily calorie intake to around 800/day, less than half the usual daily requirement for health. The replacements usually come in the form of liquid shake drinks or soups. Apart from the shake nothing else should be consumed other than perhaps mineral and vitamin supplements. I consider this approach to be a form of 'chemotherapy' for diabetes, and one which requires quite intense motivational and supportive care from a health professional. The thing is it does work for some people. Some people lose weight and do indeed see their diabetes remit. But, it is a very big ask. Lethargy and coldness are quite common side effects and a course of meal-replacement liquids is not real food. For those who reach their target weight and HbA1 level, and their VLC diet comes to an end, there is another dilemma. What next? Returning to their old diet habits will almost always be followed by a gain in weight and a relapse back into diabetes. For those who chose to adopt the Official dietary advice there is a risk that they too will relapse, because Official advice is to give large quantities of carbohydrate foods to people known to be carbohydrate intolerant. The best follow-on diet would appear to be to adopt a low-carb approach and maintain it indefinitely. So, I wonder, why not forget about starvation therapy with VLC meal replacement shakes and just go low-carb with real food from the outset?

Fasting on the other hand has a long and venerable history. "Fasting unto prayer" has been used as a religious practice across the world and throughout history, and for a very good reason. It helps clarify the mind and improves perception. In prehistoric times, fasting may not have been a lifestyle or even a religious choice, it would at times have been a harsh fact of life. Another name for it may have been a 'hunger'. We humans are adapted to function very efficiently and effectively when hungry; in times past, it drove us to hunt or forage more intently. If hunger had clouded the mind and left us listless, we would have died in lean times. In fact, hunger/fasting was probably the rule rather than the exception for many of them back then. Problem is, we modern humans have precisely the same biology as our ancestors but now live with large well-stocked fridge-freezers, cupboards full of packaged and tinned food and a convenience store on a nearby street. Intermittent Fasting and Restricted Eating it seems, are potential ways to slide our body chemistry back into a more natural and healthy *glucose-insulin-lite* mode, the one in fact, we evolved to thrive on.

Bottom line – Intermittent Fasting works for many people. People lose weight with it and say they feel healthier. It just requires some thought about how to do it, some planning as to how to make it work and how to prolong glycogen-burning and perhaps get into the fat-burning modes. The only people who it may not be advisable for are children, those with medical conditions, and particularly those on certain medications, especially medications for diabetes. They would all need to check things out with their doctor first, and good luck to them with that. Some would also include pregnant women in that list. Hmmm... it is less risky for doctors and writers to play safe. But let's face it gestational diabetes is now running at epidemic proportions too. Since 1980, when our nation's diets flipped and became low-fat and high-carb, one US study reckons gestational (pregnancy related) diabetes rates have risen 35-fold, a 3500% rise.

One final thought – can fasting be used to outweigh or counterbalance the detrimental effects of a high-carb diet? My hunch is probably not for most people. Constantly flip-flopping from high-carb to fasting does not allow the body to power itself consistently without the taint of insulin. So, having fasted, let us think (briefly) about exercise. Can you walk, run or swim yourself out of diabetes? Spoiler alert – no. But, physical activity does burn muscle glycogen, which has to be replaced. Exercise can be an insulin-sparing activity.

Table 6.2 Fasting; *à la carte*

Method	Examples	Notes
Intermittent fasting (IF)	The Fast Diet (The 5:2)	Pick two days each week and cut your intake food right down to 500Cals a day (600Cals for men). This is relative, not absolute, fasting. No requirements stated about how many meals or what sorts of foods you eat; just cut the cals on 'fast days'
	Alternate day relative fasting	Much the same as the 5:2 but done 3 or 4 days each week
Absolute fasting	The late, late breakfast	Basically, extend the period of time between your evening meal to the breaking of your overnight fast the next day. Aim for 14-hour (or more) fasts. Water is allowed
	The 8:16	Much the same as the late, late breakfast but all your eating is done over just 8 hours of the day; say between 11am and 7pm. Nil by mouth for the remaining 16 hours, though water is allowed.
	The 4:20	Much the same as the 8:16 but food is squeezed into just four hours; say from 1pm to 5pm though water is allowed at any time
	Alternate day absolute fasting	Nil by mouth every other day though drinking water is allowed
	2-, 3- or 4-day fasts	Much the same as alternate day fasting but extending the duration of each fast. Water is allowed. This method will move you into benign dietary ketosis

- There is, of course, nothing to stop one from mixing and matching. Say, 3 late breakfasts and 1 or 2 low-cal 'fast days' in a week

- It is likely that choosing low-carb foods between periods of fasting will magnify the effects of the fast and over time help correct insulin resistance

Table 6.3 Who should consider fasting? A hunch too far?

Status	Features	Dietary need
Insulin sensitive	Healthy*, normal weight	Lowish carb/Low-GI
Insulin dominated	Healthy, overweight**	Low carb/GI + IF
Insulin resistant	Metabolic syndrome***, pre-diabetes/T2DM, and overweight/obese	Strict Low carb/GI + IF

GI – glycaemic index. Low-GI basically means a low sugar, low starch type diet…basically the *Beating Diabetes* approach
IF – intermittent fasting
T2DM – Type-2 Diabetes Mellitus
* Healthy includes full blood check results being normal too (blood pressure, triglycerides, HbA1, uric acid, possibly also ultrasound san of liver and pancreas)
** Note: weight and health problems are not necessarily linked. Some people are healthy and overweight. Others have normal weight but are unhealthy. They can be TOFIs – thin on the outside, fat on the inside. Actually, recent opinion says being overweight is not healthy even if the person currently appears to be so
*** The Metabolic Syndrome is a constellation of physical and chemical disorders linked to Insulin Resistance. Various definitions exist but commonly they would include overweigh/obesity, raised blood pressure, raised glucose levels (especially fasting glucose and after a glucose drink) and raised blood triglyceride fat levels. Some also include abnormal cholesterol levels, gout, non-alcoholic fatty liver disease (NAFLD) and in women the polycystic ovarian Syndrome (PCOS).

Notes:

(1) Dr Michael Mosely investigated it in a programme called 'The power of intermittent fasting'. It was shown in the UK and worldwide on BBC TV.
https://www.bbc.co.uk/news/health-19112549

(2) *The Fast Diet* Michael Mosely and Mimi Spencer. Short Books Ltd; Revised and Updated edition (18 Dec. 2014)

Chapter 7 – Exercise

This is the shortest chapter in this book and for good reason. Type-2 Diabetes is a metabolic or body chemistry disorder and not the consequence of physical inactivity. Diabetes, say the 'experts', is about eating too much and exercising too little, gluttony and sloth in other words. I do not buy this. This is not my belief. Diabetes, or sugar-diabetes, as it used to be called, is a condition where the body has difficulty coping with carbohydrates; it's a carb-intolerance state. Exercise can be beneficial, particularly so for heart-health, no doubt about that, but the role of exercise in reversing diabetes is far less certain. That's because diabetes is a carb/insulin combination problem and unless that is addressed head-on everything else, from jogging to miracle foods, just tinkers around the edge. Diabetes and overweight/obesity aren't primarily about exercise or fitness. They are not 'walking deficiency' disorders. As the cardiologist Dr Aseem Malhotra says 'you cannot outrun a bad diet'.

However, I think just about everyone would agree that being physically active is a good thing. It is one of the most important things we can do to improve general health, boost wellbeing and protect us from a range of medical conditions. It can also be the source of much pleasure and enjoyment. So, it's official; physical activity is a good thing but, for those with diabetes, the questions are how much do we need to do, how often and why bother?

Just as with all matters dietary, there is a wide range of confusing, contradictory and sometimes alarmingly diverse opinion out there. Some view exercise and training as *the* way to health and longevity. Indeed, if he had his way, one senior public health doctor in the UK would have diabetes renamed 'walking deficiency disorder' [1]. As ever, confusing the whole issue, those with vested interests deliberately muddy the waters of truth. One soda manufacturer was recently discovered to be influencing journalists about the causes of obesity. Media delegates at a university conference went away believing that inactivity and not the sponsor's high-carb food and soda drink products, was the most important cause of obesity. Biased stories later appeared in the press, so the drinks manufacturer got what it had paid for, until it was exposed for what it was – lies.

Some people advocate short bursts of high-intensity activity, some long runs and circuits and other something far more sedate. Money can be involved too, of course. In the past, I was a member of a sports club whose slogan was 'Health and Fitness'. The assumption was that these two states were pretty much one and the same thing. In fact, I now believe it is possible to be healthy and unfit and conversely fit and unhealthy. Inevitably, is it possible to be both, or neither. The point is, being able to run a 5K or do fifty press-ups does not mean that eating a carb-heavy diet is going to be okay. 'He died in the peak of condition' is something you don't want chiselled into your tombstone.

I take the view that exercise, for me at least, should be partly recreational and partly something to help keep my body chemistry in a lean low-carb insulin-sparing mode. Not for me the agonising long jog on a misty morning, nor flailing away on those machines at the gym. I much prefer to go on frequent brisk long walks (perhaps with brief bursts of faster walking, a sort of interval training thing), to cycle if possible rather than drive, to climb stairs rather than be transported in an elevator and, perhaps, to swim a little more often than I actually manage in practice. In other words, I prefer to make my whole life physically active rather than be passive and inactive (except when I am writing books). Presently I do not engage in any sports, though I have enjoyed them in the past but I always participated for enjoyment and not primarily as a prescription for health. This is not an argument against sport, or even for flailing away on a machine at the gym. It is instead saying do sport for enjoyment and not much else. In that sense, it's a bit like eating fruit.

A much more important benefit of exercising for health and, in my view, one far more important than getting perky pecs or bulging biceps, is its glucose-burning potential. Muscles scoop glucose out of the circulation when they are working and they do it very well. In fact, the more frequently we use our muscles, the better they get at glucose extraction. The benefit for those with diabetes is that, when muscles are pulling glucose out of the circulation, they are reducing the insulin needs at the same time and less insulin is good. So, if you engage in some form of physical exercise (like a brisk walk) just before or just after a meal, some of the glucose rise the food evokes will be partially offset by the muscles replenishing their glycogen. The muscles can act like a sort of glucose-sump. Exercise, in other words, can be used as an insulin-sparing activity. So, if you do that brisk walk during a period of fasting, you nudge yourself through glycogen to fat burning that much more quickly. So, exercise will help a little bit in aiding weight loss but, I would contend that for most of us it is best done with insulin and glucose in mind, rather than about the calories the exercise might supposedly consume. Plain old exercise without dietary correction is a pretty soul-destroying way to try (and usually fail) to lose weight. It has a nasty habit of making you physically fitter whilst leaving you just as diabetic and just as overweight.

One recent development that is, quite rightly, gaining popularity is Parkrun. You can register free of charge and meet up for a 5K run (or walk if you prefer). The point is that it is sociable and there is no pressure to perform. Just turn up and go at your own pace. To find out more, visit http://www.parkrun.org.uk.

Of course, these are my personal views. They are for me and people like me. They are not for elite athletes. Those thoroughbreds live on a different plane of nutritional existence. For them, protein supplement powders and carb-loading diets may (or may not) give them a tiny edge over a competitor, an edge that can mean the difference between winning and losing. For them, fitness and that edge are the things. For me and I hope for you, health, not fitness is the goal.

So, do be active. In fact, try to be active every day. Being active can involve nothing more demanding than taking a regular long brisk walk. Actually, a short stroll is better than nothing. So, get your shoes on and open that front door but watch out for the hunger pangs that can follow exercise. It is just your body saying we have been burning glucose or glycogen and now we want to replace it. Be prepared, be aware, celebrate it but ignore it. Better to have a glass of water than a piece of cake at the end of your Parkrun.

Don't avoid exercise if you are fasting. It probably makes the fast's effects more potent but don't go mad. Modest exercise could be defined as the sort that gets your pulse and breathing rates up a bit but still leaves you able to converse without problems. Bottom line - exercise can help to prevent or reverse early Type-2 Diabetes and pre-diabetes and it can make the dietary change more effective with weight loss. However, it is only of marginal help and, for many, it isn't an effective answer. Unless the carb-insulin combo is dealt with, exercise is highly likely to fail at preventing or curing diabetes. So, do not kid yourself. Diet is the thing and you cannot outrun a bad diet [2]. Be fit *and* healthy if you can.

Notes:
   (1) Leading doctor claims Type-2 Diabetes is 'just down to laziness' **https://closeronline.co.uk/diet-body/health-fitness/doctor-sir-muir-gray-type-2-diabetes-walking-deficiency-syndrome/**
   (2) 'It is time to bust the myth of physical inactivity and obesity: you cannot outrun a bad diet' A Malhotra, T Noakes and S Phinney. http://bjsm.bmj.com/content/49/15/967?utm_content=bufferbd139&utm_medium=social&utm_source=twitter.com&utm_campaign=buffer

Part 3

I got the key to the highway
The toolkit

Chapter 8 – Change

How many low-carb dieters does it take to change a light bulb?
One, but he/she really must want to change.

A few years back, I ran a diet trial with patients of mine. It was called the ISAIAH study and was published in 2008 (1, 2). The idea was to compare how well a low-carb diet programme worked compared with the standard low-fat/low-cal diet among pre-diabetic people. It was a pilot study designed to test out the programme I had devised, rather than definitively answer the dietary question. As a matter of fact, both groups did pretty well on the programme, though the low-carb group people did better.

A key feature of the programme was not just that structured dietary advice was given, nor was it that some fun aerobics featured in each session. No, a crucial part of the programme was that it majored on how to anticipate and cope with failure. 'Don't let your lapses become relapses,' advised Maria Platts, the research nurse on the project. The part played by two other members of the team was also really important. I have to thank Dr Robert Glendenning and Professor Peter Marsh of Sheffield University for introducing me to two powerful aids to successfully achieving change. They are the Decision Balance and the Cycle of Change.

In the ISAIAH study, patients were divided into two groups. Half attended a low-carb diet themed course and the others a standard diet course. Each group had around eight members and they met six times, weekly for the first four weeks. The programme cycle ran twice, with two new groups of patients with pre-diabetes in the second cycle. Even in an average sized UK General Practice population, there was no problem finding recruits. Type-2 Diabetes, previously uncommon, is now at epidemic levels.

Each of the evening meetings lasted around 90 minutes. During the meeting, Robert or Peter spent a chunk of time with each group. Their job was motivation or, more precisely, motivation for change. One group-exercise they employed involved thinking very practically about how to change. In particular, they focused not just on the potentially good things about changing diet but also the potential downsides too. They also talked about the good things and bad things and about *not* making any changes at all. This was clever, because change to a better diet leads to two scary things, which are leaving your comfort zone and facing new challenges. A method they employed was called the Decision Balance.

Basically, they drew a big square containing four boxes on a flip-chart (see Figure 8.1). The two boxes in the left-hand column were for 'not changing' and the two in the right-hand column were for 'making a change'. In the top row, the participants listed good things; the pros, if you like. In the bottom, they listed bad things about changing or not, the cons.

Figure 8.1 Decision balance for changing from a low-fat/calorie-controlled diet to a low-carb diet

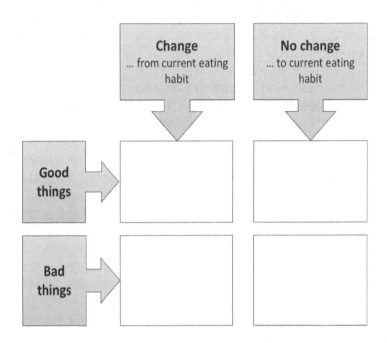

Most of us, most of the time, just consider the good things about improving our diets. We may perhaps list the bad things about the old diet that got us diabetic/pre-diabetic in the first place too but the Decision Balance chart explored the other sides to those two coins. Why not try drawing your own table and filling in the boxes either on your own or, better still, with a supportive person or even in a group? You may find it amazingly helpful. It can empower people to act when they uncover and start to understand some of their (almost subconscious) driving forces.

Figure 8.2 A completed Decision Balance chart

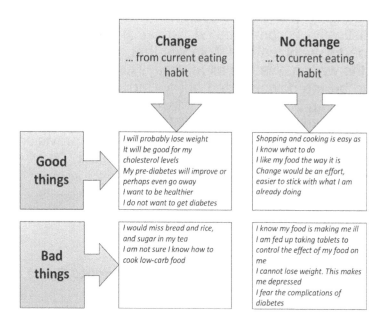

Through the 1970s, James Prochaska and Carlo DiClemente developed a structured method for helping therapists facilitate life and behavioural change with their clients. They called it the Transthoeretical Model of Behaviour Change[3]. It has been developed and modified over the years, but the underlying principle remains useful. It is still used extensively, particularly in situations where psychological or addictive issues are being addressed. Robert and Peter shared something called the Cycle of Change with the groups, an exercise which came out of the Transcultural Model studies.

When they first saw the illustration of the cycle, most of the participants remarked that instantly it made sense to them (Figure 8.3). They found it useful in identifying exactly where they were on their own personal dietary journey. Many found two of its features particularly helpful. They were that the 'Action Step' should be preceded by mindful contemplation and preparation, or getting ready to change. Rushing into change frequently fails and secondly, the cycle demonstrated, that 'Relapse' is a real and ever-present problem. It too needs to be acknowledged, addressed and put right out there in the open. Knowing that relapses can/will happen from the word go is realistically accommodated within the cycle. It makes provision for wobbles and it knows that, at times, we can all fall off the wagon. We can all relapse. The secret when we fail is not to be too downhearted but to 'move back two squares' and then jump back on again. Most people have lapses and most of us experience setbacks. Knowing stormy weather is never too far ahead should prompt us to make provision, give thought to and prepare for how we will handle it. The Cycle of Change works best when it is shared with someone who supports you and has time to talk. Again, it also works particularly well with people in groups.

Figure 8.3 Prochaska and DiClemente Cycle of Change

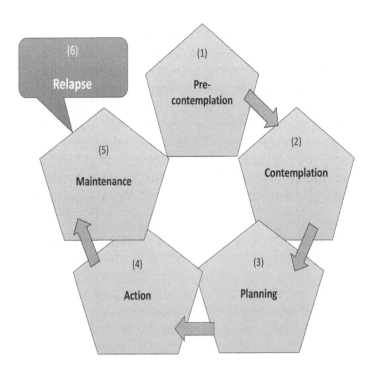

1 –   Pre-contemplation: you are not ready to change. You may not have realised that there is a problem, or feel that it isn't an important issue for you at the present time. While some in pre-contemplation may be in denial, others will know there is a problem but may decide that the time is not yet right. You may feel fine and enjoy eating all those things that are not so good for you but you are content to continue like this, at least for the time being.

2 –   Contemplation: Time to start getting ready for change. At this stage, no action is required; fools rush in… and all that but you have started to understand that there is a problem, you are beginning to get your head round it. Deciding that there is something about your diet that is dangerous, which could be improved and that change might benefit your health, does not mean you have actually changed anything... yet. However, it does mean that a light has started shining into the darkness.

3 –   Planning: A crucial stage. You are getting ready. You are preparing to make a start. You know there is a problem and you now really want to do something about it. You are approaching commitment. You have starting to consider what change will mean, how it will affect your life and how it can be done in practice. These are the Shop, Cook, Dine questions. It might mean talking with significant others in your life, or planning menus but it also means thinking about your particular vulnerabilities. It may also include drawing up a Decision Balance list.

4 –   Action: You have made that first crucial step and are now modifying your behaviour. It may be to do with alcohol, smoking or exercise, for example. It could be about making social changes in your life but it can also be about implementing a new eating lifestyle.

5 –   Maintenance: You have changed. You have done it. Well done. You are now working to sustain it in your everyday life. You will be alert for those little voices of temptation and honestly prepared to avoid lapses.

6 –   Relapse: Sliding backwards is human. You may have done very well but have now fallen back into your old ways, perhaps when you were on holiday, or was it over Christmas with its orgy of carbohydrate feasting and indulgence? Do not be afraid. You know that lapses happen; it is pretty well inevitable. So, acknowledge that this is where you are but remember Maria's advice. 'Don't let your lapses become [sustained] relapses'. Get back into the contemplation, planning and action mode and move on. This applies to small lapses as well. Confess, repent and move on.

Like the chapter on exercise, this one on change is low on word count but big on implication. I cannot commend enough spending some time writing up your own decision balance and identifying where you truly are at on the cycle of change.

Notes:
1. Can Type-2 Diabetes be prevented in UK general practice? A lifestyle-change feasibility study. Barclay C, Proctor KL, Glendenning R, Marsh P, Freeman J, Mathers N. (ISAIAH). British Journal of General Practice. December 2008
2. ISAIAH. An acronym that stands for Insulin Sensitivity And Its Applications to Health.
Prochaska, JO and DiClemente, CC. (1983) Stages and processes of self-change in smoking: toward an integrative model of change. Journal of Consulting and Clinical Psychology, 5, 390–395.
https://www.ncbi.nlm.nih.gov/pubmed/6863699

Chapter 9 – Fail

I really ought to have been a little more positive, especially so late in the book. So, let us start instead with Succeed... or perhaps How to Succeed, Despite Failures. Failure can, of course, be seen an opportunity and not just as a setback. So, let us look at what to do if you appear to be failing despite doing everything right. Who said diabetes was fair? Not me, that's for sure.

Plucking success from the jaws of defeat

- **Anticipate and plan ahead for failure.** Everyone will no doubt have their own low-carb tale to tell. Most stories will be a mixture of good and bad. Good times when things went well and less good times when they did not. Not many people will experience unalloyed 100% success, or wall-to-wall 100% failure. For most, it will be a mixture of both, hopefully more success than not. So, the first tip in succeeding is to anticipate and plan for setbacks.
- **Mind-mapping for success.** Setbacks will happen for most of us, but a bit of self-awareness will identify where your particular setback risks lurk. So, I suggest you deliberately set aside some time to think about this. Have a pen and paper handy and write down every thought that enters your head, even the whacky ones (perhaps especially the whacky ones). You can write randomly all over the page. It is better not to make it a list. Perhaps start writing the most important themes near the middle of the page. When the thoughts stop flowing, have a look at what you have got and look for any themes or areas of overlap. Circle them and connect them with lines. Keep doing this for a few minutes. This is a sort of mind-mapping exercise and can be very helpful in clarifying your thoughts and considering these will empower you to plan ahead effectively. So, a holiday in the sun with friends, staying over with relatives, eating out, the dreaded corporate buffet heaving with brown fodder; all can be minefields. Knowing and considering these in advance and giving them a little pre-emptive thought is the golden secret of success. By

the way, you can keep on adding to the map for as long as you wish as, from that map, strategies for success can emerge. Actually, sometimes they jump off the page at you. Sharing it with someone who knows you well can also be very helpful.

- **Sharing your change with others.** This can be very empowering too. It is a strategy used by many slimming clubs with great success. 'Hello, my name is Chris and I am a carb-aholic.' Yes, supportive groups can work for more than just dietary change. Smoking cessation, alcohol or substance abuse problems, driving safety awareness and even anger management interventions are often turbo-charged by group activity. Honesty is easier amongst fellow travellers on the road back from carb-ageddon. Finding a low-carb group might be a challenge but sharing things with a friend or colleague can amount to much the same thing. You may consider asking someone you trust to spare half an hour each week to listen and talk though your low-carb journey. Talking can be therapeutic and the very process of translating thought into coherent speech, slowing it down, is a curiously effective way to get your head around things. Solutions often appear as if by magic when we talk and there are numerous on-line and Facebook type forums out there.

- **We live in an obesogenic environment**. Acknowledge it and move on. A friend of mine recently told me that she had lost 35 stone in weight (around 490 pounds, 220Kg). She did not lose it in one go. Rather she lost a few pounds or a couple of stone, then put it back on and then some more. She has tried any number of diets and every single one worked well... for a while. In a disarmingly honest analytical essay she shared with me about her experiences, she identified a whole list of incidents and beliefs that consistently confounded her ambitions; life just kept on getting in the way. We now live in what some call an obesogenic environment. This means our whole lives, our services and all our interactions seem to function very smoothly when we comply with the low-fat, low-cal, high-carb norms that surround us. Life really is out to get us but why is failure such a consistent consequence of dietary change? Anticipate honestly and plan your avoidance strategies.

- **Don't let your lapses become relapses**, as Maria advised. Stuff happens but don't wallow. Get over it. Pick yourself up, dust yourself down and move on. You are engaged in a war not a battle. Actually, I don't really like military metaphors. Perhaps consider it this way instead: you have knowingly committed yourself to a better way but you are human and lapses will happen, especially when life's waters get a bit choppy.

What if things fail despite you (seeming to be) doing everything right?

Remember earlier when I said that biology was inherently variable? Remember when I said some (lucky) people can gorge on carbs and suffer no ill effects and that it was bad luck you got diabetes when annoying Mr. Lucky, didn't? Well I have a little more troubling news to share with you. There is no lower limit for carbohydrate intake below which Type-2 Diabetes is totally guaranteed to melt away. For some, a modest carb reduction is all that is needed but, for a very few particularly unlucky people whose diabetes and glucose-insulin problem is at such a pitch, almost any exposure, even the merest whiff of carbs, will keep their insulin resistance rolling on. I did tell you that life wasn't fair? Sorry no, I didn't.

So, if you have cut out sugar and cut down on starchy carbs but have not seen an improvement in either your weight, abdominal circumference, or your blood test results, what next? You may recall having seen Table 3.4 in Chapter 3 – *Shop*, the chapter about In-Foods and Out-Foods. It gives detail of the various levels of carb restriction/intake. As you can see, there are four broad categories of carb restriction.

Table 9.2 Carbohydrate intake levels

Carb content	Diet type	Approximate daily carb intake for a 2000 calorie/day diet
High-carb diet	Official Dietary Advice	300g +
Minimally reduced-carb diet	Step 1	Around 200g
Moderately reduced-carb diet	Step 2	Around 100g
Low-carb diet	Step 3	Around 50g
Very low-carb (ketosis) diet	Step 4	<30g

- There is no consensus on how to categorise quite how restricted a diet is in terms of carbohydrate content. The ballpark figures presented here are an amalgam of figures collected from a variety of sources
- The steps in the second column relate to those given in Table 3.4
- A 2,000 cal diet which is 55% carbohydrates is equivalent to around 275g carbs/day
- Phase 1 Atkins diet carb intake is around 20g/day

Conclusion

Well done for getting this far. Pat yourself vigorously on the back, or phone a friend to do it for you. I hope that all of you who try out carb-cutting will have enjoyed the change. After all, fat is your new best friend in the kitchen and fat tastes good. I hope most of you and your healthcare professionals will have been pleased with the results on your diabetes too.

Of course, for a few there will be frustration. Weight, belt size and blood results may have stubbornly stayed put for some. Actually, for some people, although weight may not have dropped, their abdominal circumference might have gone down. This is a good, if slightly frustrating, sign. It suggests that that your internal (visceral) fat is reducing, which is good and that muscle bulk from all that exercise has increased, which is also good. Perhaps for them an extra spurt of carb-cutting would produce even better results. Failing that, you may want to count your calories. Are you eating the right stuff, but just too much of it? This is more a question for those seeking weight loss rather than correcting body chemistry.

Make sure to discuss your plans and share your experiences with your health professionals. This is particularly crucial if you are on medication, which may need to be adjusted if you cut carbs or fast. They may well be signed-up believers of the Official dietary guidelines and view low-carb dining as a fad and perhaps a dangerous fad at that but they are there to advise you and you must be heard. Current official guidance for doctors and dieticians is to respect your views and opinions and to assist you in making those changes, even if they may harbour some doubts about your preferred method. Having them on side is definitely a good thing. Weighing up conflicting advice is never easy, but it is something everyone trying to dine in a low-carb way now has to put up with.

Part 4

It's the Rules

Chapter 15

The 'Beating Diabetes' Ten Commandments

The spirit is willing though the flesh is weak

This chapter is a summary of *Beating Diabetes* presented as a set of rules: the Ten Commandments. When Moses produced the originals over three thousand years ago, his followers said that they would do all that was commanded of them, although many lapsed, it seems. Each of *Beating Diabetes'* Commandments revises a particular message of the path away from insulin resistance back to normality. In this chapter, you will find all the arguments and explanations repackaged into flavoursome low-carb bite-sized chunks. Brevity means no punches get pulled. I do write with a sense of indignation that so much avoidable suffering is being caused by the very system that is charged with preventing and treating it. Instead of improving health, Official policy is one of giving in to a slow defeat. This just is not good enough, particularly when reversal of the condition can be a real possibility for so many.

The First Commandment:
If you hope to reverse your diabetes, start by ignoring the dietary guidelines*

This is quite a shocking statement to make, especially from a fully paid-up health professional like me, but I believe it to be true. Why? Well, as you now know, Official guidance bases its healthy eating advice on including plenty of carbs with every meal. The carbs they promote may taste great and we may love to eat them, but in evolutionary terms they are novel foods. They are not ones that would have turned up in nature and certainly not in the quantities and potencies that we now have to contend with today. The result: we have all now become citizens of Planet Diabetes.

Way back in Welcome to Planet Diabetes, you read about what diabetes actually is. Type-2 Diabetes is a state of insulin excess and insulin resistance. The effects of these are to degrade control of blood sugar and HbA1c levels and it can make us fat. The target of medical intervention in diabetes is to bring sugar and HbA1c levels down. Medical intervention, or drugs, as it is also called, is designed to modify the *effects* of diabetes. Medical intervention does not address the *cause* of diabetes. That is why medical interventions do not (indeed cannot) hope to reverse diabetes; its only hope is to slow it down a little. 'Once a diabetic, always a diabetic' is the Official line, a policy of defeat and acquiescence, because it pays no heed to the real *cause* of diabetes: a carb-heavy diet.

Official guidelines embrace two other major errors. Firstly, that obesity causes diabetes and secondly that dietary fat is a dangerous disease-mongering food. Wrong on both counts. Obesity, like diabetes, is caused by the double whammy of too many carbs and too much insulin and not the other way around. That is why some now use the term *diabesity,* as diabetes and obesity are just two sides of the same coin.

More on fats and oils below. In the meantime, if you want to try and reverse your diabetes, start by ignoring Official guidelines on healthy eating by cutting the carbs and enjoying the fat.

* This was also the title to Dr Sarah Hallberg's excellent TEDx talk, which can be viewed free on You Tube.
https://www.youtube.com/watch?v=da1vvigy5tQ

The Second Commandment:
Cut out sugar

At the end of the day, common or garden everyday table sugar, or sucrose, to be precise, is just a chemical. It isn't a nutrient in the way that certain proteins and fats are. As a matter of fact, there are no essential sugars or carbohydrates at all. None. Apart from newborn babies, we can all live and even thrive on a zero-carb diet. I am not suggesting you do that. It is just an interesting fact that puts the whole sugar thing into perspective.

Sucrose is the stuff we stir into tea or coffee and when we do that, we are adding sugar to our diet. We can add sugars in many other ways too. For example, sprinkling it on strawberries, eating confectionery, or drinking non-diet fizzy drinks. Sugar is added into recipes, particularly in packaged foods (read the labels). Dieticians rightly advise us to be cautious when it comes to adding sugars into our diet. Actually, I don't think they go far enough in their advice about added sugars, especially when it comes to people with diabetes, which, let's face it, is a condition driven in large measure by sugars in the diet.

Sucrose splits during digestion into glucose and fructose (fruit sugar). You really should keep the amount of anything that delivers fructose right down. Glucose is the stuff we know as blood sugar, but fructose, although chemically similar, is something else. It does not stimulate insulin release and is not metabolised like glucose throughout the body. It behaves chemically more like a fat. In anything other than small quantities, fructose can become a potent cause of fatty build-up in the liver and pancreas. This fatty accumulation is also a cause of insulin resistance.

For those of you who use the Glycaemic Index to see how carby a food is, fructose poses a problem. The GI is all about glucose; fructose doesn't figure in it at all. The result is that table sugar has about half the GI score of glucose and guess what? Food manufacturers can tout sugary foods as 'lower GI' even though this is patently ridiculous. Sugary foods like fruit get a lower GI rating than you might expect if you consult a carb-counter or calorie-counter book. Fructose just isn't on the GI radar.

Many dieticians are, however, far less concerned about limiting your intake of the sort of foods where sugars are an integral part of their make-up. Again, I am thinking particularly of fruit. Even if you refrain from dusting fruit with sugar, you will still get a significant sugar hit when you eat it. Fruits are sweet because they contain... wait for it... sugar! Sugar in fruit is a lure deployed by plants. Sugary fruit snares us into eating it and in return doing something for the tree that produced it. Modern fruit is far sweeter and juicier than any previously naturally occurring fruit ever was. Why? Because we humans have been busily engaged in genetic engineering them for millennia, we have bred the sweet and succulent qualities we desire into them. This quality, the inherent sweetness of some foods, allows devious advertisers to state that their food has 'no added sugar' or that it is 'naturally sweet'. These weasel words simply mean the stuff – fruit in yoghurt for example – contains sugar and possibly lots of it. 'We didn't add it. The fruit did, so it doesn't count'. Well guess what? It does; it counts a lot.

The *Beating Diabetes* advice about fruit, or any other food, whether intrinsically sugary or extrinsically sweetened, is to avoid it. Cut out all added sugar and minimise your intake of sweet foods, like fruit, that are 'naturally' sugary. The reason is simple. If you have diabetes or pre-diabetes, you are, by definition, someone who has a sugary and starchy carb driven problem. Unless and until you stop pouring sugar into yourself, you will not be able to reverse the condition. Yes, I know. It's unfair; life is unfair but you are where you are. Get over it – or just take the medication.

The Third Commandment:
Cut out starchy foods too

Starches are also carbohydrate foods. Unlike simple sugars, they are chains of sugars all zipped up together. This, some say, makes them complex but sadly, when it comes to digestion, they are far from complex. In fact, as far as your stomach is concerned they are simple. Starches are just pre-sugars and they too feed the flames of diabetes (pre-sugar diabetes?). For me, starchy foods are 'stealth-sugars'. So just to remind you, starchy carbs are foods made from flour and root vegetables. Bananas are starchy, an exception among fruit. Most starches come from grains or tubers.

The Big-6 carbs include five starchy foods; bread, pizza, pasta, rice and potato. Other starchy carbs include cakes, biscuits, pretzels, bagels, crisps and crackers. Starchy carbs can be sneaked into any number of other foods too. They appear as thickeners in sauces and dressings, binding agents in hamburgers and sausages and bulking agents in packaged foods, too numerous to mention.

At the end of the day, starch is just a bunch of glucose molecules. Eat starchy food and basically you are just eating sugar. Dr David Unwin and colleagues working in Southport, UK, worked out a nice way of showing just how much sugar-potential various starchy foods contained. They did this using something they called 'teaspoon equivalents of sugar' and 4g is the amount of sugar in one teaspoon. Coincidentally, 4g is the total amount of glucose the average healthy person has in their entire bloodstream. Yes, we only have around one teaspoon of sugar in our entire circulation. So, for the following starchy foods they worked out that...

- Boiled spaghetti = 3.7 TSEs/100g
- Apple juice = 3.5 TSEs/100ml
- Banana = 4.8 TSEs/100g
- French Fries = 5.0 TSEs/100g
- Baked potato = 6.3 TSEs/100g
- Basmati rice = 6.7 TSEs/100g
- Brown bread = 10.8 TSEs/100g
- Raisins = 17.0 TSEs/100g
- Coco Pops = 24.2 TSEs/100g

TSE = Teaspoon equivalents of sugar. It is about 4 grams
https://phcuk.org/wp-content/uploads/2016/06/Dr-David-Unwin-Dr-Jen-Unwin-Success-For-People-With-Diabetes-In-Primary-Care-And-Beyond.pdf
Note: some data presented here comes from Product Labels

Are you surprised? To give you some idea of what 100g is, a medium-sized apple weighs in at around 150g. If your breakfast consisted of 100ml apple juice, 30g of coco puffed rice (that's the miniscule official serving size), a small 100g banana, all washed down with a black coffee (*sans* sugar: 'hey I'm on a diet, guys'), you would have consumed the equivalent of over 17 teaspoons of sugar. Seventeen! That is the glucose hit your body would get from this apparently modest meal and that is just for breakfast. You haven't even left the house yet.

Are you shocked? If that was your breakfast, then it is no wonder you would need to make shed a load of insulin to cope with this nutritional assault. How come no one told you this before? More to the point how come our national dietary guidelines and all those armies of doctors, nurses and dieticians keep telling people with carbohydrate intolerance (diabetes) to keep eating the very foods that pour glucose into the body and then find themselves obliged to give them drugs to cope with their crazy diet?

If you have diabetes or pre-diabetes, cut the sugars, cut the starches, cut those high-carb foods right down. Indulge yourself occasionally for pleasure if you must, but do not for heaven's sake base your normal everyday diet on these foods. Sugary and starchy carbs can be occasional welcome treats but, please, not staple foods for everyday consumption.

There are of course many low-carb foods that can be eaten and enjoyed almost without limit. They are called vegetables, from asparagus to zucchini. These are the vitamin, mineral and fibre-loaded real super-foods that should form the bulk of what most goes on your plate. Yes folks, it's official – apart from the meat, fish, eggs and dairy, I am a vegetarian.

So, the third commandment is to cut right down on all those starchy carbs. Have a look at the In-Foods section in Chapter 3 for a list of the wonderful delicious foods you can enjoy instead while reversing your diabetes.

The Fourth Commandment:
Enjoy natural fats and oils

Let's face it, we have got to eat something and if grains, potatoes and sugar are out, then what else is there to dine on? Short answer: plenty. There are all those yummy vegetables for a start but there is much else besides, and one big tasty treat is the fatty foods. Actually, fat is a name straight out of a chemistry book. In plain English, by fat I mean meat, fish, nuts, olive oil, butter and even cheese. Yes, these are just some of the foods that deliver good old natural fat and much else besides. What is that spluttering noise I hear? Sounds like dieticians and guideline writers choking on their quinoa.

We humans have been dining on fatty foods forever. In fact, some human societies like the traditional Inuit peoples of the high Arctic, have lived healthily eating pretty much nothing other than fat. Fat is tasty and fat is satisfying. Start the day with a fatty breakfast (like a cheese omelette) and you will cruise way past elevenses with barely a thought for a snack. Why? Because fatty foods are filling and can keep you feeling full for several hours. They have the satiety factor. Carbs, on the other hand, burn off like chaff, leaving our stomachs rumbling after barely a couple of hours.

Surely fat is bad and even dangerous? Doesn't fat cause heart attacks? Err, nope. True, the wise men of medicine have been telling us this since the 1960s but the research they based their erroneous advice on was flawed, partial and sadly biased from the word go. Fat didn't cause heart attacks then and it doesn't do so now. Fatty foods don't make you fat either, unless you eat them with a side order of sugary and starchy carbs. It is carbs that make you fat because of the insulin they need for digestion. Remember insulin? It's the hormone of storage. It is difficult to store fat in the absence of insulin and you cannot release fat in its presence. Carbs need insulin for digestion. Even protein requires some insulin but fat doesn't need insulin at all. Fatty foods are *the* insulin-sparing foods. Fatty foods are the diabetic's friend.

148

Are all fats fine? Sadly no. Nearly everyone now knows that the trans-fats are bad. These are manufactured industrially. The process involves rearranging the chemistry of cheap vegetable oils, transforming them into solid fats. It uses heat and pressure, the presence of hydrogen gas, plus a metallic catalyst. Not something to try at home, dear reader. Trans-fats are on the way out now, and good riddance, but the oils that they are manufactured from are still with us. These are the cheaply produced, industrially extracted seed oils, things like cottonseed, rapeseed, soybean and sunflower seed oil, the so-called vegetable oils.

Vegetable oils have an aura of naturalness about them but, like their trans-fat predecessors, they are industrial products. These oils do have many culinary qualities, some are nutty, some are flavour-free and many have high smoke points but they are all high in Omega-6 fatty acids. These are classed as PUFAs, or polyunsaturated fatty acids. They differ from the sorts of fats commonly found in meat and dairy, much of which are saturates and olive oil, which is a mono-unsaturate. These so-called vegetable oils, which don't even come from vegetables, also have a nasty habit of changing their chemical nature when heated, especially if re-heated repeatedly; think chip-pan. It is thought these degraded oils could have toxic effects in the body. Want to know more? Then read Nina Teicholz' landmark book *The Big Fat Surprise*. Published by Scribe UK.

Some Omega-6 is essential for health, but we only need it in small quantities. We can get as much as we need quite naturally if our diet contains egg, poultry and nuts. In larger amounts, Omega-6s have been linked with a number of inflammatory conditions like arthritis, bowel and liver disease, heart conditions and even Alzheimer's disease. So, my view is that keeping these industrially extracted seed oils out and replacing them with naturally occurring products like olive oil, coconut oil, butter, lard and suet is preferable. Have a look at Appendix 1 for some data on oils and fats. It may surprise you. In the meantime and with the exception of trans-fats and vegetable (omega-6 PUFA) oils, celebrate the fatty foods on your menu.

Health Implications of High Dietary Omega-6 Polyunsaturated Fatty Acids. Patterson E et al. J Nutr Metab.2012; 2012: 539426.

The Fifth Commandment:
Plan your meals and write lists

Changing anything usually requires some forethought and planning if it is to be effective and, with a dietary change, you may well need to spend some time getting your head around things before you venture out shopping. Going low-carb is easy, but only if you stop to consider things first. If you don't, you may find covert carbs sneaking under your radar. The solution is to plan your meals in advance. I gave some examples of specimen menus earlier but they are just some of the foods I like to dine on. You may well have different preferences. So, plan your own sequence of meals, yes – a sequence. That way one meal may lead to the next. You may find preparation times can be reduced too.

Cookbooks are good but I find the internet even better these days. There are hundreds, if not thousands of low-carb dishes to discover. In South Africa, the low-carb approach is called Banting. William Banting, a Victorian funeral director, was one of the first to advocate successfully carb-cutting as a way to lose weight. Anyway, if you enter 'Banting meals' in a search engine, you will get more hits than you will ever need. An alternative site I visit regularly and recommend highly, for recipes and suggestions is dietdoctor.com

Planning and listing will make you more efficient when you do the shopping. You will be less likely to stumble into buying the wrong stuff. Sticking to the list will usually make shopping cheaper too. Of course you will, no doubt, be tempted when you come across apparent bargains but always ask yourself whether the bargain is on the In-Food list.

The Sixth Commandment:
Get cooking
You have planned your lovely meal. You have made a list of

the ingredients required. You have boldly cruised around the shops without wavering so now it is time to cook that meal. Yes, I know, cooking takes time. Most meals cannot be thrown into the oven without some preparation. There is just is no getting away from it. If you are going to cook from raw ingredients, it will take some effort. It is demanding. If you have no intention of cooking and do not have someone else to do the cooking for you, then I am sorry to say that you had better stay on friendly terms with your doctor. You may well be seeing a lot of each other in the next few years.

But is cooking all about tedium and drudgery? Is it just a necessary evil? I do not think so. Of course, as someone who is now in 'late middle-age', I now have more time to cook than when I was younger and worked long hours and shared responsibility for several children. There again, most people who have diabetes or pre-diabetes are also in their fifties and beyond and could make time to cook. This, sadly, is starting to change now with younger people, some of whom in their twenties, who are developing diabetes.

Cooking is work but it can be a source of pleasure with significant rewards in the pride of creation. Indeed, very few worthwhile achievements come without a degree of dedication and practice. Cooking is no exception and of, course, it can be shared with others. The secret for those fearful of cooking is to have a go and start with something simple. Prepare the same dish regularly and you will get better at it. It will become easier and the results more dependable. You can then throw in some variation and slowly expand your repertoire. Don't forget just how much help there is for you out there on the internet.

Sorry but at the end of the day, you are just going to have to go for it or risk sliding deeper into diabesity.

The Seventh Commandment:
Dine mindfully

Apologies if that sounds a bit trendy but I do believe there is a lot to be said for having a mindful approach to things generally and eating in particular. Dining is one of the crowning joys of civilized life. So many important events involve dining. We celebrate with meals. We show sympathy with food. We mark important events and milestones in life with feasts. Dining is a core component of being truly human. So how come some homes no longer have a dining room or even a table in the kitchen? I am not thinking poverty here. I am thinking about house designers who see no utility in providing a living space with a surface around which to dine. This is diminished living and it is dangerous.

Dining is not refuelling. Its focus is not the recharging of batteries and stocking up on nutrients. Dining is a social activity that brings people together around a table. Dining is a celebration of the wonder of real food and culinary creativity.

Mindless eating, on the other hand, is often about consuming cheap, salty, carb-heavy, processed and packaged foods. So often, mindless eating plunges one into dangerous eating by consuming too many of the Big-6 sugary and starchy items. Too often such food is Omega-6 fat and seed-oil heavy. Mindlessly eaten foods tend to be the ones that slide us deeper into diabetes, obesity and heart disease – even if they taste nice. The wages of mindless eating are, all too often, weight gain and diabetes, two of the so-called diseases of western civilization.

So set the table, serve the food, celebrate your meal together and thank the cook. This is dining and it is one of the keys to healthy living but don't forget about the washing up.

The Eighth Commandment:
Fast strategically

All-day grazing, from the moments after rising through to the late pre-sleep snack, is the new normal on Planet Diabetes. Many of us now power our bodies exclusively on the glucose from the foods and drinks we consume around the clock. Glucose surges into our bloodstreams at meal times and continues to trickle in between meals as we nibble and sip our way through the day. Only during our hours of sleep do we switch over to burning some of the starchy glycogen stored in our livers. Even then, we merely dip into it briefly, never enough to drain the liver's stores and so oblige us to turn to our fat stores for fuel. Yes, we live in insulin-dominated times and it is driving us into diabesity.

It need not be like this. We can switch our fuel supply quite simply. After all, there are four to choose from (food-glucose, glycogen-glucose, fatty acids and ketones) and all but one, food-glucose, burns without any need for insulin. There is much more about this in Chapter 6. Briefly, a great way to cut your insulin need and with it, your insulin resistance, is a combination of low-carb dining and strategic fasting. When you have a short fast, your insulin levels drop like a stone and you start using your liver glycogen for fuel. Actually, most of us do this every night unless we get up to raid the fridge for a snack. If you fast for around 12-14 hours, your glycogen battery will be empty and you will automatically and seamlessly switch over to burning fat. Fat gets broken down (lipogenesis) and transformed into fatty acids so if you dine early in the evening and fast through till a late-late breakfast the next day, you will end up burning fat. That is a golden double benefit; no insulin and fat burning at the same time and, if you do this often, your body chemistry will tool up and magnify its benefits. Chapters 6 and 7 also address how cunningly deployed physical exercise can turbo-charge the benefits of fasting. Indeed, this may be the most powerful positive effect of exercise in diabesity.

Fasting has been around since the dawn of humanity in various guises. Fasting was what happened during lean times when there was little food around. Remember, it sharpened our wits to hunt and gather more effectively and is a discipline still used to make prayer and meditation more powerful. Today, short but regular periods of fasting have become one of the most powerful treatments we have available to beat diabetes. Fasting can be absolute or relative, sustained or intermittent. Fasting methods can be mixed and matched but whatever method employed, the benefits accrued are the same, i.e. down-regulating insulin and switching the body into its fat-burning mode. What's not to like about fasting?

The Ninth Commandment:
Think things through

Fools, they say, rush in where angels fear to tread, so tread carefully and thoughtfully.

If trying to reverse diabetes is your desire, then stalk your prey. Think about why you want to do this, not just superficially about how good a change of diet might be. Give some consideration for a few moments to some of the awkward downsides of change. In Chapter 8, you will find two exercises that can really help with thinking things through. One is the Decision Balance, which you can use to weigh up the pros and cons of change versus no change but there is also something called the Cycle of Change. Have a look at them again. Where would you say you are right now on that journey? Both these exercises are worth doing. Many people have found doing them with others is even more helpful. It is good to talk, usually. The point is, you really do need to be a bit strategic here. You may see the benefits of changing. You may fear the consequences of not changing. You may or may not have support from family, friends or health professionals but launching yourself into change must be done at the right time, at the moment it is most likely to succeed and least likely to fail. You need to know where the sweet spot is (perhaps not the best metaphor at this juncture).

The Tenth Commandment:
Be ready for failure

Stuff happens. Two steps forward, one step back. This is what life is like. So right now, I say, anticipate failures (plural). Get ready for setbacks. They are going to happen. You may know your weaknesses and can predict where you may fall. Perhaps like me (and Lord Darlington in Oscar Wilde's play Lady Windermere's Fan) you can resist everything...except temptation. The secret is to get back up, dust yourself down and when the moment is right, return to the fold. Remember Maria's maxim? 'Don't let your lapses become relapses.' Learn from these occurrences so your risk of failure is reduced in the future. All this is discussed further in Chapter 9. Okay, dear reader, we are almost done. Just the (fascinating) appendices to go.

Part 5

The Appendices

Appendix Section

To keep the text clear and uncluttered, I have tucked a lot of data away in a series of appendices. They will enable you rapidly to check out such things as the carb or Omega-6 content of a range of foods, for example. They are arranged in groups; fruits, nuts and dairy etc.

The reason behind the selection of food groups is to clarify carb content where there is variation within a range of similar products, butter and condensed milk for example. Food groups where there is little ambiguity have not been included here for example meat, fish, confectionery and flour-based products. All meat and fish is low-carb unless processed in some way. All confectionery and flour products are high-carb. For details on these see Chapter 3 and the In-foods, Out-Foods tables.

I though some information about alcohol in its myriad alluring forms might be interesting too. The section of food labelling is a short rant on the slippery ways food producers in concert with advertisers, deceive us by stating (some of) the truth.

Appendix 1 – Fats and Oils
Appendix 2 – Nuts (including peanuts and chestnuts)
Appendix 3 – Fruit
Appendix 4 – Dairy
Appendix 5 – Alcohol
Appendix 6 – Food labelling
Appendix 7 – Diabetes drugs

Appendix 1 – Oils and Fats

Broadly speaking, oils and fats fall neatly into three groups. There are those we get from fish and animals, those simply extracted from plants and the oils that are industrially extracted from seeds. Opinions differ on which fats are good or bad, which oils are better or worse. Until the 1950s, animal fats, like butter and suet, were seen as good. Things changed when they were blamed for the rising tide of heart attacks in the United States, wrongly as it happened. Over the following two decades, longstanding food lore was turned on its head. We entered an era of low-fat, low-saturated fat, high-carb driven dietary advice. The science for this was wrong right from the beginning and the experts inadvertently gifted us with epidemics of obesity and diabetes.

My view, for what it is worth, is that simply extracted plant oils are good and animal fats may be even better. They are natural fats and oils. They are, in my view, the healthy fats and I enjoy consuming them every day. The industrially extracted seed oils are something else (and here I would also include cold-pressed, so-called 'extra-virgin' seed oils). These seed oils are usually called vegetable oils even though they do not come from vegetables. Although, from a culinary perspective, there is a great deal to commend them, they all have one big impediment – their Omega-6 fatty acid content is very high. There are also concerns that when heated during cooking, their chemical nature changes, with health-damaging implications. This appears to be a particularly issue if they are used repeatedly at high temperature.

We need polyunsaturated fats like the Omega-3s and 6s in our diet. They are both 'essential' fats. Essential means we need to eat them because our bodies cannot manufacture them and without them we get ill. In nature, the balance between these two classes of fats appears to be important. A healthy ratio of Omega-6 to Omega-3s seems to be between 1:1 and 4:1; certainly <10:1. A ratio of 50:1 is now not uncommon. The total quantity of Omega-6s consumed is also important. Why? Well, it seems consuming too much Omega-

6 fat tips the balance in the direction of inflammation within our bodies and an inflammatory regime predisposes us to a range of ailments; e.g. arthritis, heart disease, autoimmune disorders. Well, it seems consuming too much Omega-6 fat tips the balance in the direction of inflammation within our bodies and an inflammatory regime predisposes us to a range of ailments; e.g. arthritis, heart disease, autoimmune disorders. For that reason, I now strive to keep a firm lid down on how much Omega-6 I consume, and the simplest way to do that is to minimise the amount of industrially produced seed oils I use in my cooking and dining. This includes soya bean, rapeseed, rice bran and wheat germ oil. I do use some of the nut oils, despite their high Omega-6 content. However, nut oils are used in very small quantities for flavour and so seem okay to me. If I do need to use a high-smoke point oil, I use avocado or coconut oil.

Below, you will find tables giving details on a number of common fats and oils. The data was collected from a range of sources. Unearthing information about them proved surprisingly difficult. There was also quite a lot of disagreement from one authority to another over the precise figures. I suspect biological variability may explain some of this. The differences were, for the most part, quite small. I therefore present, in good faith, what appears to be a reasonable assessment but they are ballpark figures. Individual products may differ from the figures listed here.

The various fats and oils are listed in the tables in ascending order of Omega-6 fat content. So, coconut oil and butter are near the top as they have only 1-2% Omega-6 (good) and safflower oil is at the bottom as it has an Omega-6 content of 74% (bad). Interestingly, all the high Omega-6 fats and oils, from rapeseed oil down, are without exception industrial seed extracts (the so-called vegetable oils).

If you want Omega-3 oils in your diet, you won't get much from any of these fats or oils. Oily fish and fish-oil products are your best source of these 'essential' fatty acids. Flax seed might appear to be a good source but the particular type of Omega-3

---

fats it contains are not handled well by the body. Sorry, veggies, it's all about the fish.

Table A.1 Commonly used Fats and Oils. Approximate data listed in ascending proportion of Omega-6 PUFA content per 100g of commodity

	Omega-6	Omega-3	Omega-6/3 Ratio	SFA	Mono	Smoke point (°C)
Butter	1	1	1	52	21	177
Coconut oil	2	0	-	87	6	177-204
Suet	2	1	2:1	59	36	200
Beef dripping	2	0.4	5:1	51	38	210
Ghee (clarified butter)	3	-	-	51	21	252
Olive oil	8	0.7	11:1	14	76	207-242
Lard	9	0.5	18:1	40	43	182
Margarine	9	4	2:1	35	37	182
Goose fat	10	0	-	28	57	190
Palm oil	10	0.3	33:1	48	37	232
Hazelnut oil	11	0.1	110:1	8	77	221
Flax seed oil	12	53	1:4	9	20	225
Avocado oil	13	1	13:1	13	68	271
Rapeseed oil	20	10	2:1	7	59	204-230
Peanut oil	31	0	-	20	47	232
Rice bran oil	33	1	33:1	21	39	254
Sesame oil	43	0.3	143:1	15	38	210
Cottonseed oil	50	0.1	500:1	26	18	216
Corn oil	50	0.9	56:1	14	30	232
Soybean oil	52	7	7:1	16	22	232
Hemp oil	54	18	3	10	12	165
Wheat germ oil	55	5.3	10:1	19	17	225
Walnut oil	58	12	5:1	9	17	160
Sunflower oil	63	0.1	630:1	12	21	232
Safflower oil	74	0.1	740:1	10	12	266
Ghee (vegetable)	No data	-	-	47	39	252

SFA – Saturated Fatty acids
Mono – MUFAs, or mono-unsaturated fatty acids
PUFA – Polyunsaturated fatty acids (the ones that include the Omega-3s and -6s)

Data sources:
- McCance and Widdowson
  https://www.gov.uk/government/publications/composition-of-foods-integrated-dataset-cofid
- on-product data box figures
- **https://theconsciouslife.com/foods/avocado-oil-04581.htm**
- **http://nutritiondata.self.com/facts/beef-products/3478/2**
- **https://www.nutritionvalue.org/Beef%2C_raw%2C_suet%2C_variety_meats_and_by-products_nutritional_value.html**
- **https://www.nutritionvalue.org/Oil%2C_rice_bran_nutritional_value.html**

Notes:
- All figures expressed as % of 100g, rounded to nearest whole number. Figures > 1 rounded to nearest whole number
- Note that finding reliable and consistent data proved very difficult. The sources I used were at times contradictory. These figures should therefore be taken for rough and general guidance only
- The figures may not always add up to 100%. Other fats may be present in some cases
- Only animal fats consistently have an Omega 6/3 ratio less than 10:1
- Of all the industrially produced seed oils, only rapeseed oil appears to have a reasonably good Omega-6/3 fat profile. Having said that, its absolute Omega-6 levels, though lower than the other industrially produced seed oils, are significantly higher than coconut and olive oil, for example. Perhaps ghee (clarified butter) and avocado oil are better frying options
- Smoke Point. This is the temperature at which (wait for it) the oil starts to burn and make a smoky vapour. This will affect the taste of the oil and anything cooked in it. Push the temperature above smoke point and you will eventually hit flash point. This, surprise number two, is when the stuff actually starts to go up in flames. This is not good for cooking purposes. A range of smoke point figures is given for some oils. Generally, the more refined the oil the higher its smoke point is.
- Regarding calories - fats and oils are calorie dense at between 8-900 Kcals/100mls
- Special note regarding vegetable ghee, sometimes called vanaspati ghee. This is a processed vegetable product. It is made from a variety of processed seed oils, e.g. palm, sunflower, soya and cottonseed oil. Basically, it is not butter at all. It is a type of margarine. Its Omega-6 and -3 content is therefore likely to reflect those of its ingredients. Some varieties may contain trans-fats. It is widely used in India and Pakistan and also may be used in Indian restaurants in the UK.
-

Rough Cooking Temperatures
Pan fry 120C
Deep-fry 160-180
Oven bake 180C

Appendix 2 – Nuts and Seeds
True seeds and nuts are all calorie dense, around 500-750 calories per 100g. A serving size is (should be) much less than 100g, of course. Chestnuts, which are not really nuts at all, come in with fewer calories (around 170/100g). This is

because they are low in fat. They are however pretty starchy little things. Again, the quantity consumed is important. If you are on a very low-carb diet, give them a miss.

The Omega-6 content varies quite a lot, but once more the quantity consumed is important. When I make my nut-based *no-grainola*, I tend to make it almond, pecan, brazil and hazel heavy, with just a few walnuts.

Peanuts are, of course, pulses and not true nuts at all. A small number of peanuts seem fine, although they are moderately high in carbohydrates and a bit Omega-6 heavy. Sunflower seeds are, of course seeds, as are chestnuts.

This table lists nuts in ascending carbohydrate content. Cashews (which I love, salted) are, it turns out, surprisingly naughty little carb-bombs. Omit them if you are on a very low-carb diet. As a matter of fact, they are a form of fruit and not nuts.

Table A.2 Nuts and Seeds. Approximate data listed in ascending carbohydrate content per 100g of commodity

Nut	Total carbs/100g	Total protein/100g	Total fat/100g
Sesame	1	18	58
Walnuts	3	15	69
Brazil	3	14	68
Pine	4	14	69
Macadamia	5	8	78
Hazel	6	14	64
Pecan	6	9	70
Almonds	7	21	57
Pistachio	8	18	55
Peanuts	13	26	46
Cashew	18	18	48
Sunflower	19	20	47
Chestnut	36	2	3

Notes:

- Figures (mostly) rounded to nearest whole number
- Figures derived from more than one source, which explains how some figures do not add up precisely
- Omega-3 and -6 data not included. All nuts are very low in O-3 fats. The O-6 fats vary, but are a tiny proportion of total fats. Pecans and walnuts are the highest O-6 containing nuts at just 1% each
- Sunflower seeds, peanuts, cashews and chestnuts are not nuts Principal data source **https://www.gov.uk/government/publications/composition-of-foods-integrated-dataset-cofid**

Appendix 3 – Fruit

Remember my seemingly jokey name for fruit, high-fructose tree-candy? Well, the point is, I wasn't joking. Fruit is a sugar-dense food. That is why it tastes sweet and that sweetness is because it is packed with sucrose, a sugar-combo made from glucose and fructose, or fruit sugar. Starchy bananas are an exception. They liberate glucose during digestion and only a small amount of fructose. So, when you eat fruit, you are eating sugar. Some fruits are less sugar-heavy, like berries but others are very sugar-dense, like dried fruit. It will be no surprise that candied fruit and fruit in syrup are very carb-heavy indeed as they are already a sugary food with added sugar.

Fruit tastes good and, if you enjoy it, then you have a good reason to eat it. There isn't any other good reason to eat it. You will get some vitamin C and perhaps some potassium from some items but these are as nothing compared to the real super-foods – vegetables, nuts, meat, fish and dairy. So, if you want to do the 5-a-day thing, the one we have been groomed into believing for a quarter of a century, then please major, almost to the exclusion of anything else, on vegetables.

All the figures presented here are ballpark ones. No doubt there will be many exceptions like a super-sweet apple or extra-sweet raspberry. So, use these figures as an outline as they are just for guidance.

Berries

Tasty and pretty low-carb for fruit. Garnish a yoghurt or ice cream with a few berries. Those clever little berries pack more sweetness than their carb-count would suggest.

Table A.3.1 Berries. Approximate data listed in ascending carbohydrate content per 100g of commodity

Berry	Carbs/100g
Gooseberries	0
Raspberries	5
Strawberries	6
Blackberries	12
Blueberries	13
Gooseberries	13 (with sugar)

Notes:
Portion size here is crucial. For a 30g serving, the carb counts listed can be divided by three.

Whole fruit

Big fruit, big sugar. Eat them whole (with skins on for things like apples) to get the most fibre. Do not squeeze or pulp them and no smoothies, please. As with everything else, the consequences of eating these 'Almost Out-Food' depends on how much and how often you eat them.

Table A.3.2 Fruit. Approximate data listed in ascending carbohydrate content per 100g of commodity

Fruit	Carbs/100g
Lime	<1
Rhubarb	1
Avocado	2
Lemon	3
Mandarin	4
Melon (cantaloupe)	4
Grapefruit	7
Melon (honeydew)	7
Melon (watermelon)	7
Tangerine	7
Peach	8
Nectarine	9
Orange	9
Pawpaw	9
Plum	9
Satsuma	9
Pear	10
Pineapple	10
Apricot	11
Kiwi	11
Apple	12
Cherries	12
Mango	14
Grapes	15
Banana	23

Notes:
Again, portion size here is crucial. To be certain, weigh your fruit serving. Of course, having weighed it once, you won't have to do it again unless you forget. Oh, and just look at the carbs in bananas, even more than in sugary grapes.

Tinned fruits in syrup
The only surprise here is that fruit in syrup isn't even higher in carbs. Each item here is a naturally sugary fruit, preserved in yet more sugar. If you must eat them regularly, then praise the Lord and pass the medication.

Table A.3.3 Fruit in syrup. Approximate data listed in ascending carbohydrate content per 100g of commodity

Fruit in Syrup	Carbs/100g
Mandarin	13
Pear	13
Peach	14
Fruit cocktail	15
Gooseberries	16
Plum	16
Pineapple	17
Cherry	19

Notes:

- The clue is in the name syrup (sugary liquid). Fruit in juice will generally have a lower carb content than fruit in syrup

Fruit juices

Juice delivers all the sugar, from more pieces of whole fruit than you would ever eat in one go, but with a fraction of the fibre. Remember you normally only have 4g of glucose in your bloodstream. Can it be a surprise to anyone that regularly drinking 200mls of orange juice in with its sugar hit of around 18g (over four times what normally have in your entire bloodstream) is Route-One for Diabetes Central?

Table A.3.4 Fruit juice. Approximate data listed in ascending carbohydrate content per 100g of commodity

Fruit juice	Carbs/100ml	Cals/100ml
Grapefruit juice	8	41
Orange juice	9	42
Apple juice	11	45
Pineapple juice	12	51
Grape juice	15	63

Notes:

- Portion size, once more is crucial. Not many of us will be satisfied with a measly 100ml serving. Some manufacturers suggest a serving size is 150ml, which equates to a very small glass. I suspect most people will drink a 200ml serving, which for orange juice would deliver 18g of carbs or the equivalent of 4½ teaspoons of sugar. Of course, the carb in fruit and fruit juices is sugar, sucrose. That is why it is so sweet.
- The data will vary from one product to another. I took these figures from juice in cartons, all of which advised that the juice counted as one of your five-a-day fruit and veg portions.

Crystallised and dried fruit

Take some fruit, extract all the moisture and guess what? You get a concentrated sugar food. One fresh apricot may weigh 35g. Eat two (75g) and you may get 8g of carbs. Two dried apricots, on the other hand, only weigh around 12g but they give the same carb-hit as 75g of the fresh fruit. Problem is a 'serving' of dried apricots can be around seven fruits, which will give health-conscious apricot eater a 26g carb-hit.

Table A.3.5 Crystallised fruit. Approximate data listed in ascending carbohydrate content per 100g of commodity

Crystallised and dried fruit	Carbs/100g
Prune	34
Fig	53
Mixed peel	60
Apricot	63
Cherry (Glacé)	66
Date	68
Mixed dried fruits	68
Raisin	69
Sultana	69

Notes:

The crystallisation process involves desiccation (removing water) and preserving it in sugar (crystals). Although most people would not want to consume 100g at a time, these are all carb-dense foods.

Appendix 4 – Dairy

Dairy products vary widely in their nutrient qualities, ranging from almost-zero-carb butter and cream through to condensed milk, which is 56% sugar. Cheeses, too, varies in nutrient content. Although all are either low or zero carb, they are protein rich so people on a very low-carb regime would need to limit their intake. The conversion of dietary protein into glucose does stimulate some insulin release.

What headline messages do I take from the data presented? Firstly, the carb content of milk is the same whether it is skimmed or full-fat. So, from a purely carb point of view, pick the one you enjoy. The calorie content does vary, but unless you consume a large amount of milk, the extra calorie-load for choosing full-fat milk isn't huge. I have, however, swapped from double to single cream for pouring on to my modest handful of berries. The calorie difference is significant. I now reserve double cream for making chocolate mousse. Yes, I still seem to have a residual thing about calories. Actually, I prefer single cream with berries.

Table A.4.1 Dairy produce. Approximate data grouped and listed in ascending carbohydrate content per 100g of commodity

Cheese	Carbs	Calories	Fat	Protein
Feta *	0	264	21	17
Brie	0	344	28	20
Camembert	0	292	24	20
Cheddar	0	416	35	25
Parmesan	0	416	20	36
Stilton	0	412	36	24
Dolcelatte	<1	367	33	18
Feta – reduced fat	<1	103	3	19
Gorgonzola	<1	334	3	19
Cambozola	1	426	41	14
Mozzarella	1	236	18	18
Halloumi	2	336	27	21
Ricotta	3	135	11	7
Cottage cheese	4	104	6	10

Notes:
- *Caveat emptor!* These figures are approximate and for guideline information only. Different brands often have values significantly at variance with those posted above. Always read the food data table on the product package
- Most single serving yoghurt pots contain 110-150g
- Data sourced mostly from the Ocado website in 2019
  https://www.ocado.com/webshop/startWebshop.do

Table A.4.2 Cheese. Approximate data listed in ascending carbohydrate content per 100g of commodity

Cheese	Carbs	Calories	Fat	Protein
Feta *	0	264	21	17
Brie	0	344	28	20
Camembert	0	292	24	20
Cheddar	0	416	35	25
Parmesan	0	416	20	36
Stilton	0	412	36	24
Dolcelatte	<1	367	33	18
Feta – reduced fat	<1	103	3	19
Gorgonzola	<1	334	3	19
Cambozola	1	426	41	14
Mozzarella	1	236	18	18
Halloumi	2	336	27	21
Ricotta	3	135	11	7
Cottage cheese	4	104	6	10

Notes:
Some varieties contain carbs, up to 4g. Always check the package nutritional information table

- Beware crackers and biscuits for cheese. Unlike the cheese itself, they are carb-dense
- Hierarchy of data sources used:
- 1) Obtained from shop bought product information table
- 2) McCance and Widdowson's The Composition of Foods (6th Summary Edition) Published by The Royal Society of Chemistry
- 3) Carbs & Cals Pocket Counter (in association with Diabetes UK). Chris Chayette and Yello Balolia. Published by Chello.

Appendix 5 – Alcohol

Even those who never touch a drop of the stuff have to deal with alcohol. Alcohol is present in small amounts in over-ripe fruit. It is also produced by fermentation as food passes through the gut. Because alcohol is a toxic substance, we all have chemical systems standing by, ready to break it down. That standby is an enzyme called alcohol dehydrogenase (ADH) and it lives in the liver, see Figure A.5.1. As a matter of fact almost all animals and even humble bacteria, have ADH or similar enzymes. That is because nasty, lovely, toxic old alcohol is a pretty ubiquitous substance. The main reason to include a section on alcohol is that it is a food-energy source and, particularly when taken in the late evening, can delay the switch to glycogen burning and the fasting state.

Figure A.5.1 The metabolism of alcohol

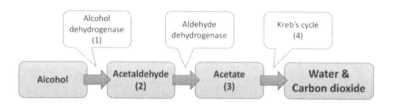

Notes:

1. Alcohol dehydrogenase is the enzyme the liver uses to break down alcohol (ethanol)
2. Acetaldehyde is the first break-down product. This is a nasty little compound that can cause tissue damage. Thankfully it doesn't last for long before it too is broken down. Vitamins C and B1 (thiamine) protect against the damaging effects of acetaldehyde
3. Acetate or acetic acid, yes vinegar. Perhaps where the phrase getting pickled comes from. This combines with Co-enzyme A and enters the...
4. ... Kreb's cycle; a series of chemical steps that generates cellular energy-storing compounds and produces water and carbon-dioxide as its end products

So, how much alcohol is in a drink? Depends on the type of drink and how much of it is consumed. Table A.5.1 gives some figures to work with. Note carefully: the alcohol content of beer, for example, can range from just over 3% to 9% so check the label. Note also that the volume you drink may differ from the examples given above. The % of alcohol is sometimes called the alcohol by volume (ABV).

Table A.5.1 The alcohol, calorie and carb content of various drinks

Drink	Given volume of drink	Typical alcohol content in UK units in given volume	Calories in given volume	Carbs in given volume *
Beer	1 pint (570ml)	2.5	200	**16-30**
Lager	1 pint (570ml)	2.5	227	**18**
Champagne	175ml	2.4	133	**<1**
White wine (dry)	175ml	2.4	115-131	**<1**
White wine (medium)	175ml	2.4	150	**5**
White wine (sweet	175ml	2.4	175	**11**
Red wine	175ml	2.8	120-133	**<1**
Rose	175ml	2.4	150	**5**
Sherry	25ml	0.5	30	**1.5-2**
Port	25ml	0.5	35	**3**
Gin/whisky	25ml	1.0	59	**<1**

* Bear in mind that 1 teaspoon of table sugar is estimated to be around 4g. So, a pint of lager could well deliver the equivalent of 4½ teaspoons of sugar. Champagne is an eminently more suitable tipple for those with diabesity.

These figures are ballpark estimates. Information sources vary widely on their figures for calorie, carb and alcohol data for very similar drinks. Serving sizes vary too. In the US, drinks come in fluid ounces. In most other places it's in mls. I have used mls with the exception of beer and lager, which are presented in UK standard pints. Pints in the US are 16 fl.oz, 20% smaller than the 20 fl.oz ones served in the UK. Confused?

There is a significant difference in carb-counts between brewed beverages like beer and lager and dry wines including Champagne. Beers and lagers contain the sugar maltose from the malt used to feed the yeast. Ciders, too, contain sugars that can come from the fruit but may have added as sucrose as well. Ciders can have a very high carb-load at up to 20g per pint. This is the equivalent of around 5 teaspoons of sugar. There are many lower-carb ciders out there that are much lighter in sugar. Unlike beers and wine, ciders often have a nutritional information box for you to check out.

I have not added data for alcopops, cocktails, Baileys, non-diet mixers, punches, mulled wines etc. etc. It should be pretty obvious by now that these are high-carb offerings that have no place in the low-carb *Beating Diabetes* approach to healthy eating.

All alcohol-containing drinks will raise blood alcohol levels. The more grams of alcohol there is in the drink, the higher blood levels will go, see Table A.5.2. The actual level will vary a little from person to person and whether it was consumed with a meal or not. The chart below gives you an idea of what a number of drinks can do to blood alcohol levels. The liver removes the alcohol at a steady rate until it is all gone. There isn't anything you can do to speed this up. Note: These figures roughly correspond to changes seen in an 82Kg person and where one drink contains 8g of alcohol. 8g of alcohol is equivalent to the UK's 1 unit of alcohol. The blood alcohol concentration (BAC) figures are rounded to 2 decimal places.

Table A.5.2 Approximate alcohol clearance times

Number of drinks (UK units)	Likely blood alcohol concentration (BAC)	Very approximate time till blood alcohol levels go back to zero (minutes)
1	0.01	60
2	0.02	120
3	0.03	180
4	0.04	240
5	0.06	300

Note: *1 unit of alcohol is equivalent to 8g of pure alcohol*

If you combine information from Tables A.5.1 and 2, you can work out roughly what effect the drink will have on your blood alcohol level. So, for example if you drink two 175ml glasses of white wine, you will have consumed 38.4g of alcohol (4.8UK units). This will raise you blood alcohol level to around 0.06mg/l and it will take roughly and on average around four and a half hours for levels to drop down to zero. If your glass is more generous or the alcohol stronger, the level will go higher and the time to complete clearance will be extended. Alcohol clearance is affected by gender, whether it has been taken with a meal or on an empty stomach and a number of other variables. When alcohol and its metabolites are present in your bloodstream, they become an energy source. Some would contend that alcohol is the fourth 'macronutrient' or food type (the others being carbs, fat and protein). Alcohol can also interfere with blood glucose levels and the way insulin works. Drinking alcohol before bed will delay your switch into liver glycogen burning mode. As you can see, having a very modest two units will result in alcohol lingering in the bloodstream for at least a couple of hours. Therefore the take away messages are...

1. If you wish to enjoy alcohol, choose low-carb alcohol drinks (Table A.5.1)
2. Keep your alcohol intake modest. Alcohol can interfere with the beneficial effects of low-carb dining
3. Do not drink alcohol late in the evening. No wine after nine is my motto.

Warning: You must not use the data presented here to work out when it might be safe for you to drive. The data presented is for general information. Many other factors can affect the rate of alcohol clearance from the bloodstream. There is nothing you can do to speed it up, but it can be slowed down. The only safe level of alcohol for driving or operating machinery is nil, zero.

Appendix 6 – Food labelling

Oh! What a tangled web we weave
When first we practice to deceive[1]

On the face of it, food labelling is a really great idea. What could be better than actually telling us, the customers, what is in the packaged food we buy[2]? I suppose to a large extent we do now get the information we need for many of the foods we buy but, in my view, this is only as long as we ignore the front of the box or bottle and go looking for the small print hidden round the back. The full information tables contain a wealth of information that has, by law, to be legal, decent and honest. So why, you may ask, have I started this section with a somewhat cynical attitude? Well, in short, it is because of what almost always features on the front of the packet to the detriment of the *actualité*.

The information tables on the back present data in two forms. Firstly, there are the Ingredients, listed and arranged in descending order of the amount the product contains. So, for example take the "Mayonnaise with Olive Oil" that featured in the recipe for Niçoise Salad (Chapter 4). The bottle led me to believe I might have been getting something resembling real mayo, you know, made with eggs and olive oil. But the Ingredient list started with "Rapeseed oil (56%)". That was a shock. Olive oil came in fifth at just 5%, just ahead of our old friend, sugar. So, fair cop. It was my own fault. I fell for the carefully crafted wording on the front of the package. Perhaps I should have thought "*with* Olive Oil" was a suspicious way to describe mayo. But it was my fault for not reading the (very) small print on the back before putting the jar onto the conveyor belt at the checkout.

The second thing you will usually find on the back of the package is the Nutritional Information Table. Real mayonnaise has a carb content of approximately nil. Had I read the small print on the product, I would have seen the carb content of what I bought was 2.3% per 100g. 2.3% might seem like a small amount but remember, true mayonnaise has no carbs in it. This was an alarm bell I ignored or missed. It was a clue to the true composition of the product. Once again, my own fault. I really should have read the information the manufacturer presented freely but very discreetly, just out of my line of sight.

But hey! Just one darn minute there. Surely the tastefully designed front of the package should have been just as honest? Well, no. The words Olive Oil were written in nice olive-green script above a picture of two nice pert and equally green olives. I think that visual image is what sold it to me. That was the money shot. I was in a hurry, but isn't everyone in a supermarket? I saw the word Olive Oil. I made an assumption and... game over. I was persuaded that I was buying a product that appeared more natural and wholesome than it in fact was. And all because of two small words; *with* and *style*. The product was in fact mayonnaise *style* dressing *with* olive oil. It was not, in fact, a true mayonnaise at all. What I got was an olive oil flavoured salad cream, 22% of which was Omega-6 oil (see Appendix 1).

The only unspun food information on the front was a lozenge-type information box telling me that 14g of the product delivered 372kJ/88kcals of energy, which added up to 4% of my daily energy requirement. Big deal. Unspun data, but of no earthly use to me whatsoever. Thanks for that, guys.

So:
Rule 1 – Read the product's full and detailed nutritional information boxes.

Rule 2 – Have a healthy suspicion of everything on the front/top of the packet. It is full-frontal advertising and may well present you with carefully selected items of truth embedded amongst words that disarm your brain (e.g. the words *style* and *with*).

Food labelling has been around in the UK in one form or another for over 30 years. It has been refined and amended several times. Currently the convention is to have five lozenges of data displayed prominently on the packaging. These should contain information on the products energy (calories), fat, saturated fat, sugar and salt content (Figure A.6.1).

Figure A.6.1 Take, for example, the data presented on a packet of basmati rice

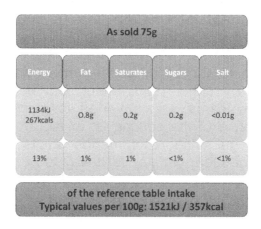

As sold 75g				
Energy	Fat	Saturates	Sugars	Salt
1134kJ 267kcals	0.8g	0.2g	0.2g	<0.01g
13%	1%	1%	<1%	<1%

of the reference table intake
Typical values per 100g: 1521kJ / 357kcal

The eye-catching stuff here is that rice is a low-fat, low-sugar product. The sellers reckon 75g is a typical serving size, so data is presented with that as the denominator. On the side of the packet, in the full Nutritional Table's 'per 100g' column, sugar is indeed listed as 0.2g but what the information on the front does not tell the person with diabetes (you, perhaps?), is that the total carb content is 77.4g/100g. Over three quarters of the product is carbohydrate. Because your Official diet guides do not admit that starch is a pre-sugar (even though that is precisely what it is), you will not realise that your uncooked 75g serving contains 58g of pre-sugar carbs. Dr David Unwin has calculated that during digestion the starch in 150g of cooked basmati rice converts to around 10.1 teaspoon equivalents of sugar, just over 40g[3]. Unwin did his calculation on boiled rice, but my package data relates to dry uncooked rice. Rice, of course, absorbs water during cooking and the cooked stuff weighs far more that the uncooked. The message I take from all this is that something quite legally promoted as a low-sugar product will in fact deliver you a ginormous wallop of sugar.

Rule 3 – Sugar is of course sugar, but starchy carbs are in effect sugars too. Starch is in a sort of pre-sugar; a stealth-sugar. So, when the package says carbs, read

sugar, because sugar is what your body thinks carbs are.

Rule 4 – Total carbs are important, but you will need to read the nutritional information box to find this out. It won't be on the front of the package.

In the rice example above, the sugar content was present as <1% of your daily sugar requirement. But because during digestion starchy carbs get converted to glucose, the true sugar consequence of the serving is, in fact, massive. Even the Official UK guidance recommends adults consume no more than 30g of sugar per day (still way too high for people with diabetes). Just one serving of cooked rice exceed this by almost 50%. Has your healthcare professional ever mentioned this to you?

Rule 5 – Because the legally required 'front of packet' information is partial, it can obscure the real sugar consequences of consuming the product.

The front of packet traffic-lights information lozenges display data for individual components of a packaged food, but not its overall advisability. Lozenges are displayed in a row but some manufacturers prefer a pie-chart approach; the so-called Wheel of Life.

Colour coding is usually added, with red signifying the nutrient is high, amber medium and green low. Some experts have criticised the whole convention as deceptive and utterly baffling to most consumers. Some information lozenges are all blue, no matter what the product contains. No food producer is going to tell you the true nutritional qualities of their packaged foods unless they are obliged to, or unless it can be spun into good news. Sadly, food producers seem to have nobbled the nutritional information requirements to their advantage, not yours. Read the full data tables and not the glossy information lozenges and wheels of life.

Rule 6 – Beware weasel words. Everything on the front of the packet is advertising. It is there to persuade you; it is

not there to inform you. *Caveat emptor.*

And just to quote one last time Michael Pollan, one of my favourite food journalists…

Rule 7 – Never eat a food that makes a health claim.
https://michaelpollan.com/articles-archive/six-rules-for-eating-wisely/

Here is a random list of words to watch out for:
- Added vitamins and/or minerals. Smokescreen for a Big-6 carb food, usually
- Beans labelled as one of your 5-a-day (it's a bean! Not a fruit or veg)
- Buttery spread. Not butter
- Cholesterol. Meaningless. Cholesterol gets broken up in digestion anyway
- Fat free. High carb (sugar or starch heavy)
- High in polyunsaturates. Full of Omega-6 industrial seed oil
- *Like*. Not what you think it is; a fake food
- Low-fat. High carb (sugar or starch heavy)
- Low-sugar. High in something else, possibly an industrial seed oil, or intrinsic sugars, or starch or any combination of the above
- Natural. As opposed to unnatural? This word can mean almost anything
- No added sugar. E.g. a fruit yoghurt where the fruit is naturally sugary anyway
- Serving size. Often the lowest amount the manufacturer can set the bar and still get away with it
- *Style*. Not what you think it is; a fake food
- Sugar-free. Artificially sweetened
- Wholegrain. Could mean wholegrain, does mean carb
- *With*. Contains a small amount of something that sounds good
- Zero trans-fat. May actually have some trans-fat in it but below an arbitrary level per serving suggestion.

Read the Information Box very closely

- As recommended by... for example, National Nutritional Organisations who would view the low-carb approach as heresy and National Medical Charities who in many instances are funded by the food industry; organisations who have sold their souls for a spoonful of sugar and betrayed us with a logo.

Notes:
1. A line from the poem *Marmion: A Tale of Flodden Field* by Sir Walter Scott
2. **https://www.gov.uk/guidance/food-labelling-giving-food-information-to-consumers**
   http://d3hip0cp28w2tg.cloudfront.net/uploads/2016-12/nutritionforncds-15-45-unwin-1.pdf

3. Appendix 7 - Drugs for Diabetes

Is it safe to go low-carb, or even fast, if you have Type-2 Diabetes or pre-diabetes? This may sound like a silly question to pose given the arguments presented so far in this book, but it is in fact a very important one.

It is generally safe to say that in pre-diabetes, and Type-2 in its early stages, a diet-change approach is an eminently suitable thing to do. However, for those prescribed anti-diabetic medication, it does need some very careful thought and professional advice beforehand. Never do this on your own. The reason? Some of the medications used to treat diabetes should either be taken with food, or should be given around meal times so that the anticipated carb-surge can be dealt with.

An example of a medicine that should be taken with food is metformin. It does not cause blood sugar levels to drop, but if you take it on an empty stomach, you could feel sick or even vomit. Metformin does not cause blood sugar level to drop, *a hypo*. An example of a medicine that must be taken around meal times in anticipation of a glucose surge into the bloodstream is gliclazide. If you take it without food, hypoglycaemia is a real hazard. Hypoglycaemia, or low blood glucose levels, can cause sweating and faintness. It could render you dizzy and unsafe to drive. It could even lead to unconsciousness; it could, in short, be very dangerous indeed. In practice, the sulfonylurea and incretin drugs, either alone or in combination with other classes of medications, are the ones most likely to cause hypoglycaemia on low-carb and fasting diets.

While some of the more common drugs used to treat diabetes do not cause hypoglycaemia, they are almost always given in combination with drugs that do. For details, see Table A.7.1. If you are on any diabetes medications it is essential to discuss things with your doctor or diabetes specialist nurse before you start diet change. This is particularly important for the sulfonylurea medicines and the injected incretins and insulins. In both cases, not only do you need to eat, but you need to eat carbohydrates in particular to avoid a potentially dangerous drop in your blood sugar levels. A change to low-carb eating would require dose adjustment and mandatory regular blood glucose check using a finger-prick blood tests or continuous glucose monitoring.

For information on fasting for those taking diabetes medicines, see Table A.7.2. The information in this table has been informed by advice given to people with diabetes who observe fasting during Ramadan. The situation with short absolute, or longer relative, fasts in people trying to reduce insulin resistance is analogous. Once again, for anything other than in very low-risk situations, like pre-diabetes or early diabetes in people not on medication, it is absolutely essential to seek medical or specialist nursing advice beforehand, and to monitor your progress closely with a finger-prick blood glucose meter or continuous glucose monitoring.

Table A.7.1 Comments on the various medications used for diabetes

Class and names of medication	Route	Fasting and hypoglycaemia information
Biguanides * • Metformin	Oral	This medicine does not reduce blood sugar levels. Instead it makes your body more sensitive to its own natural insulin. It should be taken with food. It can cause nausea and sickness if taken on an empty stomach. Hypoglycaemia risk low
Sulfonylureas *, ** • Glibenclamide • Gliclazide • Glimepride • Glipizide • Tolbutamide	Oral	These medicines increase the amount of insulin in your body. They <u>must</u> be taken with food. They can cause hypoglycaemia, particularly if your dietary carb intake is low. If the insulin secretion they evoke has no diet derived glucose to work on, hypoglycaemia is a significant hazard
Alpha-glucosidase inhibitors * • Acarbose	Oral	Slows up starch digestion so less glucose is available to be absorbed. Should be taken with food. Hypoglycaemia risk low
Secretagogues *, ** **(meglitinides also known as prandial glucose regulators)** • Repaglinide • Nataglinide	Oral	These have to be taken just before food. They can cause hypoglycaemia. Little point in using these medicines if you are on a low-carb diet as they cause a rise natural insulin secretion and work on dietary carbs
Glitazones (thiozolindendiones) • Pioglitazone	Oral	It does not have to be taken with food. Works by reducing insulin resistance. It rarely causes hypoglycaemia however it is often given in combination with other drugs that do
DPP-4 inhibitors (gliptins) *** • Alogliptin • Linagliptin • Saxagliptin • Sitagliptin • Vildagliptin	Oral	They do not have to be taken with food. They rarely cause hypoglycaemia. However, these medications are generally used in combination with other drugs and in people with significant diabetes problems. They work by keeping the incretin levels in the body up. Incretins stimulate insulin release, but only when it is needed
GLP-1 receptor agonists (Incretin agonists) *, *** • Exanatide • Albiglutide • Dulaglutide • Liraglutide • Lixisenatide	Injection	On their own, these do not often cause hypoglycaemia. However, they are generally used in combination with other drugs where hypo attacks are a very real hazard. Incretin hormones cause natural insulin secretion to increase. Incretin agonist drugs work similarly and increase natural insulin secretion when it is needed
SGLT2 inhibitors *, *** • Dapagliflozin • Canagliflozin • Empagliflozin	Oral	With water, before food or with food. Can cause hypoglycaemia when used in combination with other medications. These medications are generally used in combination with other drugs and in people with significant diabetes problems. They cause glucose to flow out of the body into the urine
Insulins **	Injection	Dose and food intake need to be carefully matched. Hypoglycaemia is a significant risk. Insulin treatment works by bringing blood glucose levels down

* Medicines that should not be taken on an empty stomach
** Medicines that can cause hypoglycaemia (low blood sugar levels)
*** Medicines that do not cause hypoglycaemia on their own, but can do in combination with other anti-diabetes medicines
DPP – Dipeptidyl peptidase. GLP – Glucagon Like Peptide, also known as Incretins. SGLT – Sodium-glucose co-transporter

Table A.7.2 Fasting recommendation in diabetic people during Ramadan

	Low risk	Moderate risk	High risk	Very high risk
Diabetes state	For healthy people already deploying lifestyle measures. HbA1c <7%	Same as low risk but HbA1c 7-8%	Hyperglycaemia, HbA1c 8-10%, not for the elderly, those living alone, with diabetes complications, or with other significant medical conditions	Severe hyperglycaemia, hypoglycaemia in last 3 months, HbA1c >10%, not for the elderly, those living alone, with diabetes complications, or with other significant medical conditions, pregnancy or dialysis
Medication	Metformin, Alfa-glucosidase inhibitors, or Glitazone	Same as low risk	Same as Moderate risk but using Sulfonylureas, Secretagogues, Gliptins, Incretin agonists, SGLT2 inhibitors, or Insulin	Same as high risk
Fasting advice	Fasting generally fine	Fast with caution	Probably best not to fast	Do not fast

Notes:
- For anything other than low-risk people who are not on medication, the involvement of a health professional is crucial
- NB Insulin injection therapy is not mentioned here but doses would need to be carefully monitored and adjusted during carb reduction or fasting. This is something that absolutely must be done in concert with a health professional
- Data here adapted from an algorithm chart in the paper 'Recommendations for management of diabetes during Ramadan: update 2015'. Ibrahim M et al. **http://drc.bmj.com/content/3/1/e000108**

Figure A.7.1 Where drugs work in treating diabetes

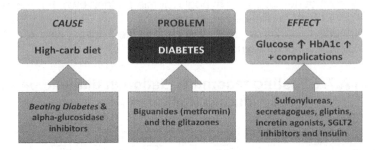

Notes on how these interventions work:

Low-carb *Beating Diabetes*Reduces glucose with diet change

Alpha-glucosidase inhibitors	Reduces dietary glucose uptake from the gut
Metformin	Improves insulin sensitivity so natural insulin works better
Glitazones	Reduces insulin resistance so natural insulin works better
Sulfonylureas	Increases insulin within the body
Secretagogues	Increases insulin within the body
Gliptins	Increases incretin activity which increases insulin within the body
Incretin agonists	Increases incretin activity which increases insulin within the body
SGLT2 inhibitors	Promotes dietary glucose loss into the urine
Insulin	Increases insulin within the body

Glossary

5-a-day – The "5-a-day for better health" slogan, conceived in 1988 by The Californian Department of Health Services, took off in 1991 when it was endorsed by the Produce for Better Health Foundation, an advocacy organisation for the fruit and vegetable growers of America. Currently, the UK's NHS advises we all eat five 80g portions of fruit and vegetables each day. The foods should be made up from five different foods. The *Beating Diabetes* approach is to support 5-a-day but only if at least 4 are all true vegetables. Any fruit you eat should be whole and unprocessed so no juices or smoothies.

Big-6 – A shorthand reminder of the main Out-foods (See Tables 3.2 and 3.3 in Chapter 3). The Big-6 are bread, pizza, pasta, rice, potato and sugar. Note, five are starchy foods and one sugary. Food groups not included in the Big-6 are meat, fish, dairy products, vegetables, nuts and pulses.

Carbohydrate – The three main food types are fats, proteins and carbohydrates (the macronutrients). Some would now add alcohol as a fourth major food type. Carbohydrates (carbs) are further divided into sugars, starches and fibrous foods. The only pure carb we regularly eat is table sugar (sucrose). All other cabs incorporate some fat and protein as well, to a lesser or greater extent. In *Beating Diabetes*, carbs generally means foods high in sugar or starch (like bread, pizza, pasta, rice and potato), which liberate glucose during digestion.

Carb-insulin combo – A shorthand way of saying that sugary and starchy foods, which raise blood sugar during digestion, raise insulin levels too. Eat carbs, make insulin.

Carb-insulin lite – A shorthand way of saying that a low-carb food or meals (e.g. salad vegetables, an omelet) has little effect on blood sugar levels and therefore little or no effect on insulin levels.

Carb-intolerance – A condition where the body has problems dealing with the blood sugar rises that follows eating sugary or starchy foods. Type-2 Diabetes is a carb-intolerant condition.

Calories – A scientific term. One calorie is the amount of energy required to raise the temperature of one gram of water by 1° Celsius at a pressure of one atmosphere. One kilocalorie (or Calorie; note, this one has a capital c) is the energy required to cause the same shift in temperature for 1 Kg of water. One kilocalorie is what we mean when we talk about calories. It is also known a *food calorie.* The word calorie is used with its commonly accepted lay meaning in this book i.e. it means Calorie or food calorie.

Causation/association – Technical terms. Causation means that something definitely causes something else. For example, having a shower causes your hair to get wet (assuming you have any). Association means two things appear related, but one does not necessarily cause the other. For example, playing darts is associated with drinking beer. But playing darts does not cause one to drink beer. The difference may seem like hair-splitting, but it is not. When it comes to diet research, the difference is crucial. Many associations are, in fact, just random occurrences, linked only by chance. Unfortunately, most diet research is about associations, which many people then assume (wrongly) equals causation. Food research reporting in newspapers and the media almost always fails to distinguish association from causation too.

Cognitive dissonance – A psychological term. It describes the simultaneous holding of two opposing ideas. For example, wanting to protect the environment and yet choosing to go on long-haul flights (*mea culpa*). Or knowing that sugary and starch foods cause large blood sugar rises, and yet advising people with diabetes to base their meals on these very foods. Cognitive dissonance can cause stress.

Cycle of change – A way of looking at how behaviour can change over a period of time, for example, choosing to try out the *Beating Diabetes* approach. The cycle includes such stages contemplation, action and relapse. See Chapter 8.

Decision balance – Another way of analysing behaviour change. For example, cutting out sugar, or stopping cigarette smoking, which may have positive benefits, but it will also have negative aspects too. It's about the pros and cons of change. The Decision Balance also enquires about change, but also about not changing too; e.g. continuing consuming sugar or smoking cigarettes. Like the Cycle of Change, it is a very powerful way of working out how and when to make changes. It is even more powerful when done with a group of people. See Chapter 8.

Diabesity – A term coined by the late diet guru Dr. Robert Atkins. It is a word combining diabetes with obesity; two conditions that are strongly "associated" but in fact "caused" by something else (clue: a hormone made by the pancreas).

Diabetes – A collection of conditions where the body has problems processing glucose (blood sugar). Typically, glucose levels run high. Other problems can follow depending on the type of diabetes.

Type-1 diabetes. This occurs when the insulin producing cells in the pancreas stop working and there is no insulin response to a high blood glucose level. Grossly elevated blood-glucose levels, dramatic weight loss, thirst and passing copious quantities of urine are the classic signs of the condition. If untreated, it can progress to coma and death quite quickly. Type-1 typically occurs quite suddenly in children and adolescents. Type-1 is a hormone deficiency state (insulin is a hormone). The treatment is hormone (insulin) replacement therapy. Getting insulin doses right requires care and professional assistance.

Pre-diabetes. A situation where the body is not coping so well with its blood glucose levels. Glucose levels may run high, or it may take longer to clear glucose from the bloodstream after a meal, or both. Given time, most people with pre-diabetes will progress to Type-2 Diabetes as pre-diabetes is just a stage on the journey. With dietary change, many people with pre-diabetes can reverse the condition and become 'normal' again. Pre-diabetes is defined in terms of fasting and 2-hour post-load glucose levels (the glucose tolerance test).

Type-2 Diabetes. This happens when fasting or post-load

glucose (following consumption of a measured amount of glucose) levels, or both, run consistently above certain arbitrary levels. Increasingly, the HbA1c test is being used to determine whether you have pre-diabetes or Type-2 Diabetes itself. Early on, Type-2 is characterised by a combination of having excessive amounts of insulin in the bloodstream combined with an impairment of the body's response to insulin (hyperinsulinaemia and insulin resistance in medical parlance). Later on, insulin levels drop though the insulin resistance remains. These insulin derangements can also cause overweight and obesity. Note: obesity is not the cause of diabetes, it is merely associated with it. Type-2 is a carbohydrate intolerance condition, one where the body is no longer able to deal efficiently with sugary and starchy carbs. Removing these foods from the diet can ease and, in some cases, reverse Type-2 Diabetes. That is what this book is about. Type-2 is the form of diabetes associated with macro- and micro-vascular complications (see below).

Gestational diabetes (GDM) is usually pretty much the same thing as Type-2 Diabetes, but it only comes on in pregnancy. It almost always appears to clear up completely after delivery. I say 'appears' because in fact the body chemistry changes that are typically present before Type-2 develops will be present before pregnancy and continue after childbirth. Pregnancy, with all its hormonal changes, merely reveals the problem, for a while. Most women with GDM will go on to get Type-2 Diabetes unless they modify their diets. They are, after all, already on the journey. The shame is that when women with GDM get better after childbirth, everyone breathes a sigh of relief and nothing usually gets done. GDM is the wake-up call where everyone keeps pressing the snooze button.

LADA (latent autoimmune diabetes of adults). It is becoming increasingly clear that some people get a form of Type-1 diabetes well into adulthood. The insulin cells in their pancreas stop working, resulting in insulin deficiency. The cause is most often an autoimmune disorder; their own antibodies have damaged their pancreas. The medicines usually used in Type-2 don't work. These people generally need insuliin injections. Type-1.5 diabetes. See Double diabetes.

Double diabetes. A term that has been around for a while but not understood by many. Basically, it describes someone with Type-1 diabetes who, because of their diet, now has Type-2 as well. Typically, people with double diabetes have had Type-1 for a while, are overweight, have a carb-heavy diet and will have noticed their insulin injection doses have been creeping up. Those who move from Type-1 to Type-1.5/double diabetes are at increased risk of the vascular complications associated with Type-2 Diabetes.

MODY (Maturity Onset Diabetes of the Young). A genetically inherited form of diabetes. Production of insulin by the pancreas is affected and usually becomes a problem during the twenties. Diabetes medications, often including insulin, are usually recommended.

Diet – A little word with so many meanings and connotations. 'Your diet' is what you choose to eat. 'A diet' on the other hand is an eating programme or set of rules. People may 'go on a diet' to improve their heath or appearance. The problem is, when 'diets' come to end, they are often followed by *getting back to normal* and the regaining of all that lost weight. If this is done repeatedly it is called yo-yo dieting. *Beating Diabetes* advocates a permanent change of eating habits. It aims to become your staple-diet rather than just be a temporary-fix-diet. Below are some of the 'diets' or eating styles mentioned in this book but first, a word of caution. If you have a medical condition or are on any prescribed medication, particularly diabetes medications, you should discuss things with your usual healthcare professional before embarking on any dietary change.

Diet, The 2:5 diet – Dr Michael Mosley and Mimi Spencer's Intermittent Fasting-type diet. Cut calories, two days each week, down to just 500 (600 for men). It's a partial fast involving less food, not no food. It doesn't specify what to eat, just how much to eat. It seems to work by regularly switching the body chemistry from its usual food-burning mode to its lower-insulin fat-burning mode. It advises fasting, not starvation. It works for many people. See

Chapter 6 – Fast.

Diet, The 8-hour diet - Another Intermittent Fasting approach. Only eat during an eight-hour period each day. This extends your natural overnight fast to 16-hours. It is not about calories. It is about switching energy sources within the body from food through glycogen to fat burning. See Chapter 6 – Fast.

Diet, A balanced diet – A phrase often used by Official diet and medical experts, but rarely defined. I take it to mean a low-calorie, low-fat, low-saturated-fat, low-salt, high-carb, high in wholegrain, high in fibre, 5-a-day way of eating, you know, the one that got you fat and diabetic in the first place. In contrast, *Beating Diabetes* advocates a low-carb approach because balanced diets seem to make so many of us diabetic and then keep us diabetic.

Diet, The Banting diet – William Banting, an obese Victorian funeral director, was the first great public proponent of low-carb eating. It worked for him and he told as many people as he could about his secret of success when he published his *Letter on the Corpulence.* Today, in South Africa particularly, the word Banting is used to describe low-carb dining.

Diet, Ketosis diet – If you choose to eat very few if any sugary or starchy foods, then your body will use fat to generate power. This can be fat from your meals or fat from your fat stores (adipose tissue). If you follow this eating lifestyle and are modest with your portion sizes, the fat liberated from your body-fat stores will be converted by the liver into something called ketones. The body can motor along very nicely burning ketones instead of glucose indefinitely. Indeed, before farming was invented ten thousand years ago, our hunter-gatherer forebears would have been in a state of dietary ketosis for most of the time. It is what we have evolved to do. You can see if you are in ketosis by testing your urine with ketone dipsticks. Keto diets appear to be good for those wishing to lose weight and reverse their diabetes.

Diet, Low-cal – There is something attractive about the simple calories-in, calories-out, energy-balance way of thinking about food and losing weight. Such a shame that it

doesn't work for so many of us. When we cut calories, our bodies have a habit of moving the goalposts as our metabolic rates go down. We start to run on a fuel-economy mode and, if we keep on cutting down calories, we can force our bodies into starvation mode. The seminal work on prolonged low-cal dieting was done in the 1940s and was called *The Minnesota Starvation Experiment*. Zoë Harcombe's blog is excellent.
http://www.zoeharcombe.com/2009/12/the-minnesota-starvation-experiment/

Diet, Low-carb – Okay, you can eat as many green vegetable-type carbs as you like, but to be low-carb, you need to minimise or exclude sugary and starchy carb foods (See Chapter 3 – Shop). Starchy and sugary foods cause blood sugar levels to rise, a lot. This causes insulin to rise, a lot. Insulin promotes fat storage and blocks fat release. It makes you fat and keeps you fat. Oh, and it promotes Type-2 Diabetes too. So eschew those sugary and starchy carbs to help lose weight and prevent diabetes.

Diet, Low-fat – Fat has more calories weight for weight than protein and carb foods and so (the logic goes) it must make you fat. This simple solution to a complex problem is wrong, as is often the case with simplistic approaches. Obesity and diabetes are hormonal disturbances, not energy balance problems. Cut fat from your diet and invariably the carbs on the plate increase. When dietary advice in the 1980s told us to eat less fat, what we did was eat more carbs. There was no alternative so what we got instead were the twin pandemics of obesity and diabetes. Low-fat advice usually cautions against consuming saturated animal-type fats and promotes vegetable (industrial, seed) oils in their place. The *Beating Diabetes* approach begs to differ. It has no problem with dining on saturated animal type fats but big issues with the industrially produced seed-oils. See Chapter 3 – Shop.

Diet, The Mediterranean diet. The Mediterranean countries are the ones that surround the Mediterranean Sea. If you start in southern Spain and move clockwise around the Sea you will pass through France, Italy, Greece and the Greek islands, Turkey, Syria, Lebanon, Israel, Gaza, Egypt, Malta, Libya, Tunisia, Algeria, Morocco and Gibraltar. Portugal is traditionally included too. There is no one single 'diet' or cuisine that covers this large and culturally diverse set of countries and so there is by definition no such thing as *the* Mediterranean diet. Having said that, the term Mediterranean diet is generally thought to imply one that has plenty of vegetables, fruits, pulses, nuts, fish and unsaturated fats like olive oil. It is usually considered to be low on meat. Very unhelpfully, the NHS adds that it should also feature plenty of starchy foods like bread and pasta and it promotes vegetable (seed) oils too. Not so Mediterranean. *Beating Diabetes* is perhaps more truly Mediterranean, culturally speaking, in that it promotes shopping for fresh produce, cooking from scratch and mindful approach to dining – with minimal sugars and processed grains and the exclusion of modern industrial vegetable (seed) oils. For those looking for an Italian-style Mediterranean diet approach, Malhotra and O'Neill's *Pioppi Diet* (Chapter 3, Note 3) is perhaps one of the best around. See Chapters 3 – Shop, 4 – Cook and 5 – Dine.

Diet-heart hypothesis – This theory was the brainchild of an American physiologist called Ancel Keys. He investigated the causes of the heart-attack epidemic, mainly affecting affluent middle-aged men, that plagued the United States in the 1940s and 50s. After a visit to Italy, he quickly became convinced that cholesterol was responsible and that diet choices were to blame. In 1953, he revealed his diet-heart hypothesis to a very sceptical world. Red meat, cheese, lard and eggs, he contended, were causing America's heart-attack problem. In one bound, he leapt from hunch to total certainty and, as an afterthought, decided to look for some evidence to support his opinions. He was it turns out, wrong. Tragically and completely wrong but so persuasive was he that almost singlehandedly he embarked his nation and then the world, on its current low-fat path to diabesity. He conflated associations into causation and stands accused of cherry-picking data to suit his hypothesis. The diet-heart-hypothesis sadly is still alive and well today. It has become dogma, it's the Official view and has driven generations into believing fats are bad and carbs are by default good. It has maimed and shortened lives on a massive scale. It has been a disaster.

Eatwell plate – A pictorial representation of the Official diet of the UK and elsewhere. The US had their food pyramid, but the UK had its plate neatly divided to advise how much of various food types we should be eating. It is the diet-heart-hypothesis on a plate, literally. If *Beating Diabetes* had a plate, it would not be the Eatwell one.

Euglycaemia – A medical term meaning that blood glucose levels are in the normal (Goldilocks) range, not too high, not too low.

Fasting, Intermittent Fasting (IF) – A fast is a period of time when someone chooses to either eat less than usual, or indeed to eat nothing at all. Intermittent implies that the fast is time-limited thing. IF is not starvation. The 2:5 diet and the 8-hour diet (mentioned above) are examples. They are not designed to calorie-restrict, although fewer calories may be consumed during fast days. Rather they influence the body's choice of fuel. Rather than burning sugars from the last meal, those who fast are likely to burn body fat. Insulin levels are very low during periods of fasting. See Chapter 6 – Fast and Starvation below.

Fatty liver and fatty pancreas –Two things drive our bodies to store fat in the liver and pancreas: insulin resistance and fructose. Both have their own glossary entries. Storing fat within the liver or pancreas is not a good thing. It interferes with the function of the organs. It can also cause inflammation, which can lead to worsening of diabetes and may lead to cirrhosis and even liver failure. So, if your ultrasonographer says your liver is 'bright' or your doctor says it is fatty, think about a low-carb approach which majors on reversing insulin resistance and advises avoidance of fructose-containing foods and drinks. The abnormally stored fat in the liver and pancreas can usually be dispersed quite quickly with a very low-carb diet and is aided by intermittent fasting too. Drugs to 'treat the problem' are on the horizon.

Glucose – A simple sugar. It is the same thing as 'blood sugar'. It is one of our body's natural fuels. We have around 4g of glucose circulation in our bloodstream, though it goes up when we eat certain foods. When glucose and fructose combine, it gives us sucrose, which is the white stuff we stir into our tea, sprinkle on our strawberries and scoff when we eat confectionery. Fructose is much sweeter than glucose. Sugary foods release glucose and fructose during digestion. Starchy foods release glucose alone, because starch is a 'glucose polymer', a chain of zipped-up glucose molecules.

Glycogen – The body stores glucose by zipping it up into long chains called glycogen. Glycogen is a sort of starch. Glycogen is stored in muscles ready to liberate extra fuel when needed. It is stored in the liver too. Liver glycogen is what keeps glucose levels up overnight when we sleep and during short periods of fasting.

Glycogenesis – A scientific term. It describes the formation of glycogen from glucose.

Glycogenolysis – A scientific term. It describes the breaking down of glycogen to liberate glucose.

Gluconeogenesis – A scientific term. It describes the formation of glucose from something else in the body. Mostly it means the formation of glucose by breaking down protein, either from the diet or body structures (e.g. in starvation).

Glycaemic Index (GI) – A scientific term for a system ranking foods in their ability to raise blood glucose levels. The higher a food's GI, the higher a given amount will raise blood sugar levels. There are difficulties with the GI approach. Firstly, measuring the quantity of any given food used to calculate its GI is not straightforward and depends on something called the available carbohydrate within the food. Secondly, because virtually no fructose sugar converts to glucose during digestion, all sugary foods have a lower GI than one might expect. For example, the GIs of table sugar (sucrose), white bread and glucose are around 65, 75 and 100, respectively.

Thirdly, GI calculations do not always equate with portion sizes. For these reason *Beating Diabetes* is based more on the absolute quantity of carbs in a food portion or meal.

Glycosylated haemoglobin – Haem is the iron-containing pigment that makes blood look red and globin is the protein that carries the haem around. The protein part reacts with glucose in the bloodstream. In technical terms, glucose glycosylates haemoglobin. The more glucose there is in circulation, the more the haemoglobin gets glycosylated. The amount of glycosylation can be measured using the HbA1c test. Results give an impression of what glucose levels have been like over the last 2-3 months, which is useful for monitoring how one's diabetes control changes over time.

HbA1c – See glycosylated haemoglobin.

High-fructose corn syrup – An industrially produced caloric sweetener. Corn is macerated and treated to transform its starch into glucose. The glucose liquor is then chemically treated to transform it to fructose. The fructose is then cut with liquid glucose. The proportions of fructose to glucose will determine how sweet the syrup will be. The usual ratio used in carbonated soda beverages is HFCS 55:45, not very different to the 50:50 ratio of sucrose, but just that little bit sweeter.

High-fructose tree candy – My facetious alternative name for fruit. Why is fruit so sweet? Because it is packed with sucrose which, of course, is half fructose. Eat fruit, eat sugar. Eat lots of fruit, eat lots of sugar and get lots of insulin.

Hyperglycaemia – A scientific term. It describes the condition or state of having a blood glucose level above a certain cut-off level. We all get a 'reactive' hyperglycaemia after eating a sugary or starchy food. In diabetes, hyperglycaemia can become persistent or 'chronic'.

Hypoglycaemia – A scientific term. It describes the condition or state of having a blood glucose level below a certain cut-off point. It can happen mildly and quite naturally an hour or two after eating a sugary or starchy food. The insulin response can push glucose levels down too rapidly and the levels can swing below normal. Hypoglycaemia can also happen in those with diabetes, particularly Type-1s on insulin therapy and Type-2 taking certain diabetes medicines. A mild hypo can cause one to feel faint, sweaty and unwell. A severe hypo can lead to unconsciousness and can be a very dangerous complication.

Insulin – A natural hormone made in the pancreas gland and secreted into the bloodstream when glucose levels rise. Its job is to restore blood glucose levels to normal (euglycaemia). In prehistoric times, insulin would have been needed when honey or fruit were on the menu, which was not often, perhaps a few times a year. Today, with our sugary and starchy carb-based diets, we need insulin to do its job many times every day. Insulin performs its glucose-regulating job by transforming glucose into glycogen and when the glycogen stores are full, transforming all the remaining glucose into fatty acids. There are moved into our body fat store (adipose tissue) for storage. Fatty acids will not be released from adipose tissue if there is any insulin around as insulin blocks its release. It is difficult to store fat in the absence of insulin. You cannot release fat in the presence of insulin. Insulin can make you fat and it keeps you fat but insulin isn't the problem. It is merely the body's natural response to eating in a way that pumps high levels of glucose into the bloodstream during digestion – sugary and starchy carbs are, in other words, the problem.

Insulin domination – In *Beating Diabetes*, this phrase means that one's food and drink choices are high in sugary and starchy carbs, therefore one's body chemistry is dominated by the hormone insulin. There are two consequences. First, because insulin is the hormone of storage, someone whose chemistry is insulin-dominated is more at risk of being overweight. They usually find weight loss difficult too. Second, excessive and persistent insulin excess can lead to insulin resistance.

Insulin resistance (IR) – A situation where the body cells that usually respond to insulin get less sensitive to it. To bring glucose levels down, higher than normal amounts of insulin are required. A contributing factor to IR is fructose, a very sweet sugar found in table sugar, cakes, confectionery and fruit. It can promote fatty liver change, which in turn is linked to IR. IR is not good. It is a key driver for developing Type-2 Diabetes. IR remains in advanced diabetes despite falling insulin levels. The opposite side of the IR coin is insulin sensitivity.

Insulin response, cephalic – When glucose levels rise, so does insulin but even before a sugary food is swallowed, the body can begin to secrete insulin in anticipation. It's thought that when a sweet taste sensation from the mouth is registered in the brain, it tells the pancreas to start work quickly to prepare for the expected glucose surge.

ISAIAH – An acronym. It stands for Insulin Sensitivity And Its Applications to Health. The ISAIAH Project is the name I have given to the studies and enquiries I have conducted into diet, health and diabetes.

Ketones – A scientific term. It simply describes a group of chemicals that can be made by the liver from fatty acids. Ketones show up naturally when the glucose supply is low and glycogen stores have been used. Low-carb diets, fasting and starvation will cause ketones to appear. The making of ketones from fatty acids is called ketogenesis. They are also formed in diabetic ketoacidosis.

Ketosis – A scientific term. It describes what happens when the body is being fuelled by fat breakdown products called ketones. One of the liver's jobs is to make ketones when the supply of glucose has run low (low-carb dining for example) or if the body is unable to use glucose (Type-1 Diabetes). Ketosis can be normal (dietary ketosis) or a highly abnormal and dangerous (diabetic keto-acidosis). These are two very different things, confusingly with similar names.

Ketosis, normal – Sometimes called benign dietary ketosis. We humans probably spent most of our time in ketosis before farming was invented. Without ketosis, we would have died out as a species. Today, we can choose to be ketotic by minimising our consumption of sugary and starchy carbs and deploying the occasional fast. See Chapter 6 – Fast.

Ketosis, abnormal – Sometimes called keto-acidosis or diabetic ketoacidosis (DKA). This is a severe metabolic disturbance with a real risk of coma and even death. Benign, it isn't. DKA was often the first sign of Type-1 diabetes in children. It is also an occasional severe complication of established Type-1. It can also happen in Type-2 but usually only when certain diabetes medicines are being taken. DKA and benign dietary ketosis might sound similar, but they are in fact two very separate and distinct conditions.

Keto-diet – You can push yourself into benign dietary ketosis by cutting down severely on sugary and starchy carbs, especially if you also deploy strategic periods of fasting. There are many online forums dedicated to keto-dieting. *Beating Diabetes* may suggest keto-dieting for some, but most will do just fine by restricting sugary and starchy carb intake.

Keto-adapted – Our bodies can function indefinitely and very nicely, powered by ketones. However it can take a few days, or sometimes weeks, for the body's cells to tool up with the right enzymes for ketosis to run smoothly. Once established, ketones can become the main fuel source and keep the body functioning effectively indefinitely.

Keto-flu – Some keto-dieters find that during their very first few days in ketosis, they feel a bit lethargic. Once the body adapts, the flu abates. It appears consuming a little extra salt can help.

Lipogenesis – A scientific term. The formation of fat from glucose. Lipogenesis is one of insulin's main jobs. Lipogenesis is what is happening when we convert surplus glucose into fat and store it in our fat cells (also known as gaining weight).

Lipolysis – A scientific term for the breakdown of fat. It produces fatty acids and glycerol, the small carbohydrate molecule that usually carries fatty acids around. Lipolysis is what happens when we use our fat stores to provide energy (also known as losing weight).

Metabolic Syndrome – A medical term. Originally described by Dr Gerald 'Jerry' Reaven in the 1980s and called Syndrome X. The Metabolic Syndrome now describes a cluster of conditions that tend to travel together. They include raised blood pressure, overweight/obesity, raised blood glucose and raised triglycerides and cholesterol. Gout and gallstones are also included by some. It has become apparent that the underlying problem is Insulin Resistance. It is strongly linked to Type-2 Diabetes, stroke, heart attack and thrombosis. Official UK advice blames it to a large extent on obesity (i.e. obesity causes obesity?) but it's insulin resistance that is the driver here. Much of *Beating Diabetes* is about reversing or side-stepping insulin resistance (with low-carb dining) and with it the metabolic syndrome too.

Official Dietary Guidance – The foundations of most Official dietary guidance are that weight and calories are directly linked and that animal fats cause heart disease. It is therefore a low-cal, low-fat, low saturated fat, wholegrain and starchy carb promoting, fruit promoting diet. Basically high-carb and low-fat. *Beating Diabetes* contends otherwise. The *Beating Diabetes* approach is a low-carb, higher-fat, vegetable-loving, fruit-light approach to eating that aims to minimise glucose and insulin surges and reverse insulin resistance.

Omega-3 and Omega-6 fatty acids – These are the main polyunsaturated fats and are found in things like the so-called vegetable oils and oily fish. Fish like salmon, tuna and mackerel are rich with O-3 oils. O-6 rich foods are mainly the industrially extracted seed oils e.g. oils from rape, sunflower, cottonseed. Both O-3s and -6s are classed as essential oils. This means that they are essential for health but are not manufactured within the body. They have to be obtained from food. In nature, the Omega-6/-3 ratio is usually between 1:1 and 10:1. In modern processed foods, the ratio can be much higher, even approaching 50:1. This is a problem because O-6 oils promote an inflammatory state within the body. Many illnesses are inflammatory in nature, so trying to restrict O-6 oil consumption seems reasonable and is in fact promoted in the *Beating Diabetes* approach. For further details, see Appendix 1 – Oils and Fats.

Overweight/obesity – The conventional idea says being overweight is the result of a simple imbalance involving too many calories in, too few calories out, or both (CICO). The *Beating Diabetes* approach sees overweight and obesity as a hormonally driven disorder, the hormone in question being insulin. Convention advice to the overweight is to eat less and exercise more. *Beating Diabetes* recommends reducing sugary and starchy food consumption in order to switch off the body's hormone of storage: insulin. Within reason, calories are irrelevant for low-carb diners.

Pancreas – An organ that sits at the back of the abdominal cavity. It has two main functions. It produces digestive juices that it pours into the upper part of the bowel through the pancreatic duct after meals. It also produces hormones to regulate glucose levels in the bloodstream: insulin and glucagon. If the insulin-producing cells in the pancreas stop working, the result is Type-1 Diabetes. Early on in Type-2, the too much dietary carbs make the insulin-producing cells work excessively keeping insulin levels abnormally high.

Paradigm – A neat little word that sums up a group of thoughts, concepts, ideas and assumption about a subject. So, the Official dietary guidance paradigm is one based on energy balance and fatty food restriction. The paradigm shift that is *Beating Diabetes* contends that obesity and Type-2 Diabetes are carb-food-driven hormonal disorders. Sugars and starches and not fatty foods or the energy balance, are the problem. The paradigm for many people has started to shift.

Parkrun – Exercise is good for us, but how can we do it in an enjoyable and sustainable way and, importantly, a way that is achievable for a couch potato? Parkrun has been the answer for many. It's a 5k run or walk done regularly each week in the company of supportive and non-judgmental fellow 'runners'. Check out the link to see if there is one near you. **http://www.parkrun.org.uk**

Processed food disease – A catchphrase invented by Dr Robert Lustig, a Californian paediatric endocrinologist. It succinctly describes the underlying problem driving so many of us to overweight and diabetes. Processed foods are frequently carb and Omega-6 heavy, salty edible substances that raise blood glucose levels dramatically and yet fail to satisfy our appetites for very long. The core of the *Beating Diabetes* approach is different. It espouses a Shop-Cook-Dine approach to healthy real-food eating.

Proteolysis – a technical term meaning the breakdown of protein, sometimes to generate glucose (gluconeogenesis). We can do this with protein from our food. It also happens during starvation, but in that scenario, it is structural body proteins (like muscles) that get changed into glucose to generate energy.

Saccharine and Saccharin – Saccharine is an old word used to describe something that is sweet or oversweet. Before industrial chemists invented non-caloric sweeteners, the word was often used about sugary foods. When a certain chemist produced benzoic sulfimide from coal tar extracts in the 1870s, he was surprised to notice just how sweet-tasting it was. He patented its production, capitalized and gave it the name *saccharin*. The product fell out of favour in the 1970s because of its bitter aftertaste and a probably spurious health scare about it. Since then, many other non-caloric sweeteners have been developed, e.g. aspartame.

Starvation – Not to be confused with fasting, which is either intermittent, short-lived or both. Starvation is a condition caused by eating too little food to sustain a healthy body. Starvation has been used successfully as a kick-start to weight-reducing diets, often advising a prolonged 5-600 calorie per day intake and often in the form of liquid shake drinks. When starvation is prolonged, the body will use its own proteins to make glucose (gluconeogenesis). This will lead to muscle loss. It will also slow down its metabolic rate. Starving people feel cold and lethargic and they often develop obsessions with food. The classic Minnesota Starvation Experiment was conducted in the 1940s by Ancel Keys and colleagues (the same guy who came up with the Diet-Heart Hypothesis, see above). The physical and psychological effects observed over six months in a group of young healthy male subjects were devastating. As I mentioned earlier, Zoë Harcombe's blog on the subject is excellent - http://www.zoeharcombe.com/2009/12/the-minnesota-starvation-experiment/

Starch – Technically speaking, starch is a polymer of glucose. Starch and starchy foods like bread and potatoes may not taste sweet, but, during digestion, the polymer chain is quickly unzipped to release glucose. Most starch is made by plants and stored either in grains or underground in tubers. Because starchy foods liberate glucose and therefore stimulate insulin secretion, they can be part of the underlying problem driving obesity and diabetes. See 'stealth sugars' below. A form of starch is made in the animal bodies (including humans) to store glucose for when needed. It is called glycogen. Muscles and particularly the liver, store glycogen.

Sugar – There are in fact many sugars out there. The simple sugars include glucose, fructose (fruit sugar) and galactose (milk sugar). Double-sugars are formed when two sugar molecules are joined together. They include sucrose (glucose-fructose), maltose/malt (glucose-glucose) and lactose (galactose-glucose). Sugars occur naturally in certain foods, e.g. fruit, honey and breast milk. Today most sugar comes from sugar-cane, sugar-beet and from industrially processed corn.

Sugar, Blood – Another name for glucose. It comes either from the food we eat, from the glycogen we have stashed away in the liver, or it gets made from protein. Although glucose can be converted to fat, fat cannot be converted back to glucose in any meaningful amount

Sugar, Glucose – The basic sugar we rely on as fuel for the body. It comes from sugary and starchy foods in the diet or from liver glycogen stores.

Sugar, Fructose – Also known as fruit sugar, fructose in nature mostly comes combined with glucose as sucrose (table sugar). Fructose is sweeter than glucose. In the body, it is converted into a form of fat. Fructose does not raise blood glucose levels (that is why the GI of sucrose is lower than many would have expected). During our hunter-gatherer years as a species, fructose would have been a rare sweet treat and one that helped us store a little fat for lean times ahead. Today we are awash with the stuff and it is one of the main drivers for fatty liver disease.

Sugar, HFCS – High-fructose Corn Syrup. Corn is a starchy grain. It can be 'digested' industrially to yield glucose, which can be chemically converted to liquid fructose. Fructose can then be cut with liquid glucose to produce 'corn syrup' or as it is sometimes styled 'corn-sugar'. The sweetener used in many cola drinks is 55:45 HFCS, 55% fructose, which is just that little bit sweeter than regular sucrose.

Sugar, Sucrose – Also known as table sugar. A double-sugar molecule made from glucose and fructose. Although the culinary qualities of sucrose are significant, in susceptible people it contributes to the hormonal drive into obesity and diabetes.

Sugar, Lactose – A double-sugar molecule made from glucose and galactose. It is the sweet stuff in milk and other dairy products. Cheeses and creams contain very little lactose. In nature, lactose is the special sugar in breast milk that babies thrive upon.

Sugar, intrinsic – This describes sugars that are naturally part of a food. For example, an apple has intrinsic sugar, as does most if not all other fruit but, at the end of the day, intrinsic sugar is still sugar. A common health promotional phase used by food manufacturers is 'no added sugars'. What this usually means is that the food is sugary, but the sugars in it are intrinsic to it one of its constituent parts, e.g. cherries in yoghurt.

Sugar, extrinsic – This describes sugars that are added to a food. For example, sugar on strawberries or sugar added as an ingredient in BBQ sauce. Extrinsic sugars are the ones Official diet guidelines sometimes advise people avoid consuming. The *Beating Diabetes* approach is less nuanced. It just advises avoiding all sugars, intrinsic or extrinsic.

Sugar, Teaspoon Equivalent – Many foods that push glucose into our bodies during digestion are starchy not sugary. People often do not realise that if they eat a slice of bread, a bowl of cereal, or a serving of boiled potatoes, they are in effect consuming sugar. That is because starchy carbs are made of glucose. Even though they do not taste sweet, they are a hazard for many of those with weight problems or diabesity. Dr David Unwin, a UK GP, came up with a way of explaining it: the Teaspoon Equivalent (TSE). One teaspoon delivers 4g of sugar. It turns out that in a supposedly healthy breakfast of 100ml apple juice, 30g of coco puffed rice (that's the miniscule official serving size) and a small 100g banana, you would have consumed the equivalent of over 17 teaspoons of sugar. This would be considered healthy for diabetic people according to the Official guidelines. For more information visit **https://phcuk.org/wp-content/uploads/2016/06/Dr-David-Unwin-Dr-Jen-Unwin-Success-For-People-With-Diabetes-In-Primary-Care-And-Beyond.pdf**

Stealth-sugar – This term is sometimes used to describe 'intrinsic sugars'. Sometimes it describes sugars added to processed foods during production but, for me, the stealthiest of sugars are the starchy foods. The ones the front of packet food labels do not describe as sugars which, within minutes of being eaten, become sugar in the body (glucose). I'm thinking bread, pasta, pizza, rice and potato.

Sweetener, caloric – Another name for sugar. Actually, there are probably over 50 names for sugar out there. Truth without clarity seems to be crucial when marketing many processed foods.

Sweetener, non-caloric – These are all the zero-calorie sweeteners. The original was benzoic sulfimide (saccharin). Today we commonly eat and drink products sweetened by acesulfame, aspartame, sucralose and many other chemicals. Stevia differs in that it is a chemical harvested from nature rather than synthesised in a factory. Are non-calorics safe? The jury is still out, I think. However, one has to be suspicious when ingesting something that isn't a real food. Of further concern is that simply having a sweet taste in the mouth can push insulin levels up. See above: insulin response, cephalic.

Trans-fats – The first trans-fats were made by chemically altering cheap seed-oils like cottonseed oil. The result was a hard fat, solid at room temperature. At first, they were used as inexpensive alternatives in soap and candle manufacture, but quickly it became apparent that they could be made edible too. So, industry started spinning straw into gold and we got vegetable shortening and margarine. Trans-fats were used in any number of baked goods and packaged foods. It was the food industry's fat of choice. Making trans-fats is an industrial process. Oils have to be heated under pressure and in the presence of metallic catalysts for hydrogen to be incorporated into the structure of seed-oils. Although these products are cheap and have long shelf lives, they have bad effects on health. They increase the risk of heart disease.

Vascular – An anatomical and medical term to describe the circulatory system in the body. It comprises arteries, arterioles, capillaries, venules and veins. Most of the complications of Type-2 Diabetes are vascular

Macrovascular – To do with large blood vessels like arteries. In diabetes, macrovascular complications are ones affecting the blood supply to the heart muscle, the brain and the legs. The complications are respectively heart attacks, strokes and gangrene in the toes/feet/lower leg.

Microvascular – To do with small blood vessels like capillaries. In diabetes, microvascular complications are ones affecting the blood supply to the eyes, kidneys and nerves. The complications respectively are vision loss, kidney failure and numbness, tingling and nerve pains.

Vegetable oils – A rhetorical question: how come these 'vegetable' oils are not obtained from vegetables? Who first decided to call oils extracted from seeds *vegetable* oils? Possibly the first product to be extensively marketed was cottonseed oil. Rape/canola, sunflower, safflower, soya and corn oil soon followed. Not one of these is a vegetable. In the past, many of these oils were hydrogenated to make them solid at room temperature and with a long shelf life. Many. These were the trans-fats. Producing seed oils is an industrial process and the product, unlike butter and lard, is an oil high in pro-inflammatory Omega-6 fatty acids. The *Beating Diabetes* approach advises using other oils in cooking even though the culinary qualities of some seed oils are undoubted. See Appendix 1 – Oils and Fats.

Walking deficiency disorder – A senior doctor working for a UK government health agency famously described Type-2 Diabetes as a walking deficiency disorder. The implication is that you get diabetes by being lazy and not active enough. This advice does of course sit very comfortably with the calories in/calories out paradigm that views diabetes as the consequence of two of the deadly sins of old, sloth and gluttony. It has led to the crazy notion of adding information on how much exercise needs to be done to offset the calories in something like a bar of chocolate. It ignores the hormonal nature completely. Remember, *it's all about the insulin, stupid*. The *Beating Diabetes* view begs to differ. Its paradigm is that diabetes is the result of a diet driven hormonal disorder involving insulin. It also believes that you cannot outrun a bad diet. See above – processed food disease.

Made in the USA
Middletown, DE
19 September 2020